The Neuropsychology of Dementia

The Neuropsychology of Dementia

A Clinician's Manual

Simon Gerhand
Hywel Dda Health Board, NHS Wales

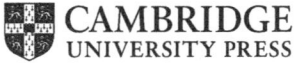
CAMBRIDGE
UNIVERSITY PRESS

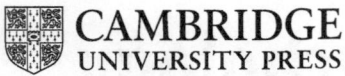

Shaftesbury Road, Cambridge CB2 8EA, United Kingdom

One Liberty Plaza, 20th Floor, New York, NY 10006, USA

477 Williamstown Road, Port Melbourne, VIC 3207, Australia

314–321, 3rd Floor, Plot 3, Splendor Forum, Jasola District Centre,
New Delhi – 110025, India

103 Penang Road, #05–06/07, Visioncrest Commercial, Singapore 238467

Cambridge University Press is part of Cambridge University Press & Assessment,
a department of the University of Cambridge.

We share the University's mission to contribute to society through the pursuit of
education, learning and research at the highest international levels of excellence.

www.cambridge.org
Information on this title: www.cambridge.org/9781009012348

DOI: 10.1017/9781009025911

First published 2024

A catalogue record for this publication is available from the British Library.

A Cataloging-in-Publication data record for this book is available from the Library of Congress.

ISBN 978-1-009-01234-8 Paperback

Contents

Preface vii
Acknowledgements viii

Section 1 Essential Background Knowledge

1 **Overview** 1

2 **Diagnosing Dementia** 15

3 **Functional Neuroanatomy** 34

4 **Neuropsychological Assessment in Dementia Diagnosis** 45

Section 2 Diagnosing Different Types of Dementia

5 **Alzheimer's Disease** 59

6 **Vascular Dementia** 74

7 **Lewy Body Dementia, Parkinson's Disease and Parkinson's Dementia, and Parkinson's Plus** 86

8 **Frontotemporal Dementia** 105

9 **Alcohol-Related Brain Damage** 121

Section 3 Intervention

10 **Cognitive Rehabilitation** 131

11 **Pharmacological Interventions** 139

12 **Reducing Risk Factors for Mild Cognitive Impairment and Early Dementia** 148

Section 4 Recent Developments/Contemporary Issues

13 **Biomarkers and Imaging** 159

14 **Dementia and Mental Capacity** 165

Index 179

Preface

The understanding of dementia has increased enormously over the last few decades. Our knowledge of the causes, accuracy of diagnosis, strategies for prevention, and treatment possibilities are all very different from where we were at the start of the 21st century. Whilst there are many excellent journals and books available to convey the latest scientific developments in the field, there is often a delay before research impacts upon clinical practice. The aim of this book is to provide a resource for clinicians, rather than academics, working with dementia, both those practising and those in training, which summarises where things are now and indicates where things are going.

Whilst the title was chosen because the book is written from the perspective of a clinical neuropsychologist, it is aimed at all professionals working in this area of health care. Although there is a theme of neuropsychology running throughout, the book also aims to also cover areas other than psychology that are necessary to understand and to work with dementia.

My decision to write a book was largely driven by two factors. The first was the need to deliver training to all manner of healthcare professionals, including but certainly not limited to clinical psychologists. I have often been asked if there was a textbook which covered all the relevant material. The second factor was supervision sessions with other psychologists, where I was asked if the information imparted in those sessions was written down anywhere. The answer was 'yes, it is, but not all in one place'. This book aims to address that.

Acknowledgements

There are many people from whom I have learned and from whom I have received support during the writing of this book. On a professional level, I must thank the team of which I am part in the NHS, particularly my learned psychiatrist colleagues: Dr Mandal, Dr Salil, and Dr O'Connor. Our Memory Assessment Service lead, Gemma Emile; our advanced nurse practitioners, Kate Bevan-Smith and Aimee Williams; and our older adults manager, Neil Mason. I am very grateful to those who have worked as assistant psychologists with me, as learning is always a two-way process. Please accept my apologies that there have been too many of you over the years to thank individually. For taking care of my health, and keeping me alive over the last few years, I am indebted to the NHS haematology departments in Cardiff and Swansea, and the bone marrow transplant team in Cardiff. For helping me to counterbalance work with other aspects of life, my thanks go to Master Leigh, Master Trudgill, and Master Nicholas. Thanks also to Andrew Vidgen and Francis Taylor, for being such loyal friends across more decades than any of us care to acknowledge. Most importantly, for giving me a reason to keep going no matter what, I thank my beloved wife Sina and my wonderful children, Laurence and Antonia.

Overview

What Is Dementia?

Dementia is a syndrome referring to a (1) *progressive* decline in cognitive abilities from a previous level, which is (2) greater than would be expected as a result of normal ageing, and (3) impacts upon day-to-day function. There are a number of different underlying pathologies giving rise to dementia, which can present in various ways, but these three elements must always be present. The other key feature is that the underlying pathologies are *neurodegenerative*, which means their effect arises from the loss of brain cells (DSM-V; American Psychiatric Association (2013); ICD-11, World Health Organization (2018)). Although a number of different conditions can affect cognitive function, including mental health problems (e.g. MacQueen & Memedovich, 2016; McDermott & Ebmeier, 2009), acute illnesses (Kalish, Gillham, & Unwin, 2014), and infections (Kukreja, Günther, & Popp, 2015), such conditions would not be considered dementia as the effects on cognitive function are potentially reversible with appropriate treatment and they do not arise from the progressive loss of brain cells. Cognitive impairment which has arisen as a result of damage to the brain from illness or injury would also not be considered dementia as the effects are not progressive, and indeed there is often a considerable of recovery of function (e.g. Chen, Epstein, & Stern, 2010; Giraud et al. (2018); Nudo 2011).

How Common Is Dementia?

When considering how common a particular disorder may be, two statistics are considered: prevalence and incidence. *Prevalence* is the total number of cases within the population at any given time point. *Incidence* is the total number of new cases diagnosed within a particular time period, usually a year. For example, NHS (2020) statistics indicated that 470,292 individuals in England had a coded diagnosis of dementia (prevalence). As part of the Cognitive Ageing and Function Studies, Matthews et al. (2016) found that, in the United Kingdom, there were approximately 210,000 new cases of dementia per year (incidence); 74,000 men and 135,000 women. The World Alzheimer Report 2015 (Alzheimer's Disease International, 2015) estimated that there were 46.8 million people worldwide living with dementia at that time (prevalence), with 9.9 million new cases each year (incidence).

Another way of looking at prevalence is to consider the percentage of the population living with the disorder. Prince et al. (2014) reported that 7.1% of people aged 65 or over have dementia, and 16.7% of people over 80. There are also a significant number of people with a degree of cognitive decline that is not severe enough to constitute dementia. This is known as mild cognitive impairment, and affects 15–20% of people over the age of 60 (Petersen, 2016).

Diagnosis of Dementia and Dementia Subtypes

Dementia diagnosis has been strongly influenced by the criteria described in the fourth edition of the *Diagnostic and Statistical Manual of Mental Disorders* (DSM-IV) (American Psychiatric Association, 2000), which required a deficit in (1) memory and (2) at least one other cognitive function to be present. Whilst these criteria may have been suitable for diagnosis of Alzheimer-type-dementia (the most common form of dementia), they are problematic for other forms of dementia where memory may be relatively spared until the more advanced stages of the disease. DSM-V has replaced the term 'dementia' with 'major neurocognitive disorder' (MND), and now places more emphasis on differential diagnosis of the individual subtypes. It should be noted that 'major neurocognitive disorder', perhaps somewhat confusingly, also covers a number of presentations which are not dementia. A deficit in memory is now no longer required as a core criterion for all dementias. DSM-V has also incorporated the term 'mild neurocognitive disorder', similar to the concept of 'mild cognitive impairment' (MCI) (Petersen et al., 1999), which represents an earlier prodromal stage of a degenerative neurocognitive condition, in recognition of the fact that an illness may have been developing for some time before it reaches sufficient severity to be considered a dementia. However, whilst MCI/MND confers a greater risk of developing dementia, this does not always occur, so the diagnosis of MCI/MND does not require evidence of ongoing decline. The individual should also be able to continue to maintain their level of day-to-day function, albeit sometimes with increased difficulty. Table 1.1 summarises the differences.

Once a likely diagnosis of dementia has been agreed, a consideration of potential causes is undertaken to identify the subtype. Although there are many possible subtypes (more than 200, according to Dementia UK), and prevalence rates can vary to some extent, there is a general consensus regarding which are the five most common types. These are Alzheimer's disease, vascular dementia, mixed dementia (which usually refers to the relatively common co-occurrence of Alzheimer-type and vascular pathology), dementia with Lewy bodies, and frontotemporal dementia (of which there are several variants). The Alzheimer's Society website lists several less common causes, stating they account for less than 5% of cases (www.alzheimers.org.uk/about-dementia/types-dementia/rarer-types-dementia#content-s tart). This means that 95% of cases seen will fall into one of the five categories listed earlier. Each of these presentations will be considered in detail in subsequent chapters.

Table 1.1 Similarities and differences between dementia/major neurocognitive disorder and mild cognitive impairment/minor neurocognitive disorder: DSM-V

Dementia/major neurocognitive disorder	Mild cognitive impairment/mild neurocognitive disorder
Evidence of a decline in cognitive ability from previous levels	Evidence of a decline in cognitive ability from previous levels
Two or more aspect of cognition affected	One or more aspects of cognition affected
Evidence of continued decline required	Evidence of continued decline not required
Decline in cognitive ability is sufficient to interfere with day-to-day function	Individual is able to continue with day-to-day function
Cognitive deficits cannot be explained by other presentations (e.g. depression)	Cognitive deficits cannot be explained by other presentations (e.g. depression)

Diagnosis will be arrived at based on converging evidence from different sources of information, including the perceptions of patients and relatives, medical investigations such as appropriate neural imaging and physiological tests, assessment of the person's level of functioning, and cognitive testing. It is often the case that not all sources of information are consistent and a definitive diagnosis can only be given post-mortem, hence the inclusion of the word 'probable' in many diagnostic protocols (e.g. the NINCDS-ADRDA criteria for Alzheimer's disease; McKhann et al., 1984). This may change with continuing development in the technology of biomarkers (McKhann et al., 2011) and neural imaging (Fox, 2019; Laforce et al., 2018; Roy et al., 2016). Despite a great deal of optimism in relation to the possible use of such new technologies, it should be borne in mind that there can be a considerable delay between the introduction of cutting-edge technology in research settings and its widespread use in clinical practice.

Toxic Agents

A common theme with all degenerative forms of dementia is the action of a toxic agent: something which is resulting in the death of brain cells. Whilst the toxic agent is present, brain cells will continue to die and the disease will progress. Any effective treatment for dementia will need to either remove the toxic agent or neutralise its effect. In order to completely reverse the effect of dementia, it would probably be necessary to regenerate brain cells in addition to neutralising the toxic agent, which is not currently possible. For most forms of dementia, we do not currently have treatments which can do either.

Let us consider an example of where there is a progressive decline in cognitive function, but where it is possible to remove the toxic agent. Alcohol-related brain damage (ARBD) is an umbrella term that includes Wernicke–Korsakoff syndrome and alcohol-related dementia (Ridley, Draper, & Whithall, 2013; Sachdeva et al., 2016). The toxic agent in these cases is alcohol, and whilst the person continues to consume alcohol their cognitive decline is likely to be progressive. However, there is a crucial difference between ARBD and most *true* dementias in that it is possible to remove the toxic agent. With abstinence from alcohol, not only does the progressive cognitive decline cease, but there is often a considerable recovery of function (Bates, Bowden, & Barry, 2002; Goldman, 1983). Admittedly it is not quite that simple, as cases of ARBD often have a second toxic agent in the form of thiamine deficiency which can cause irreversible damage. However, there is both an established and a growing evidence base for pharmacological treatment with thiamine also leading to improved cognitive function in such cases (Day et al., 2004; Thomson et al., 2002).

For most forms of dementia, the toxic agent is something which develops internally and for which we do not currently have an effective treatment. As with ARBD, there may be more than one toxic agent at work, but in most common forms of dementia the accumulation of an abnormal protein is implicated (proteinopathy). The exact mechanism by which these proteins bring about cell death may not be entirely clear, but their presence in the brains of individuals with dementia has consistently been demonstrated at post-mortem examination. This will be considered in more detail in subsequent chapters (see, e.g. Chapters 5, 7, and 8). Table 1.2 lists some forms of dementia and the associated abnormal protein.

When looking at Table 1.2, it is immediately apparent there is some overlap in the abnormal protein seen in different dementias. You might therefore ask why, if the same protein is involved, do the dementias differ? One answer is that the same protein can go

Table 1.2 Different forms of dementia and associated proteinopathy

Illness	Associated protein abnormality
Alzheimer's disease	Beta amyloid (Glenner & Wong, 1984; Selkoe & Hardy, 2016)
	Tau (Binder, Frankfurter, & Rebhun, 1985; Kankaan et al., 2015)
Frontotemporal dementia	Tau (de Silva et al., 2006)
	TDP–43 (Neuman et al., 2006)
	FUS (Nolan et al., 2016)
Parkinson's disease	α-synuclein (Spillantini et al., 1998)
Lewy body dementia	α-synuclein (Trojanowski et al., 1998)
Progressive supranuclear palsy	Tau (Cervós-Navarro & Schumacher, 1994)
Huntington's disease	Huntingtin (MacDonald et al., 1993)
Creutzfeldt–Jakob disease	Prion (Bessen & Marsh, 1992; Collinge et al., 1996)

wrong in different ways. For example, tau protein abnormalities are associated with a range of at least 20 different disorders, known collectively as tauopathies (Delacourte, 2001). Both frontotemporal dementia and Alzheimer's disease are included under this heading, and it is indeed the same tau protein which goes awry. However, (1) the mechanism by which the tau protein goes awry differs, and (2) the ensuing death of neurons is concentrated in different brain areas (Avila et al., 2006; Delacourte et al., 1998). Abnormal collections of α-synuclein protein known as Lewy bodies are considered to be the hallmark of both Parkinson's disease and Lewy body dementia (Spillantini et al., 1998); however, in the case of the former, Lewy bodies are predominantly concentrated in subcortical areas, whereas in the latter they are distributed throughout the brain, including the cortex (Gibb, Eseri, & Lees, 1987).

Mixed Dementia

One of the challenges associated with making an accurate diagnosis of dementia subtype is that comorbidity (multiple toxic agents) is not uncommon. For example, Lim et al. (1999) found that 45% of cases of Alzheimer's disease also had significant vascular pathology. A long-running study by Schnieder et al. (2007) found that only 30% of people with signs of dementia had Alzheimer's disease alone. Alzheimer's disease with vascular lesions was seen in 42% of cases, and 16% had Alzheimer's disease with Parkinson's disease. It is also worth bearing in mind that both vascular and Alzheimer-type lesions accumulate as people age without necessarily leading to dementia. Schnieder et al. (2007) also reported autopsy examinations of older people who did not have dementia at the time of death, which showed that 24% had the hallmarks of Alzheimer's disease and 18% had vascular lesions.

One reason why risk factors for vascular disorders (e.g. stroke, heart disease) are also risk factors for multiple forms of dementia caused by another toxic agent may be because there is an *additional* loss of neurons due to vascular lesions. It is also possible that vascular lesions increase the production of abnormal proteins, and vice versa.

Risk Factors and Protective Factors

In general, there is not considered to be a single cause for most forms of dementia, and even in cases where there is one clearly identified causal factor, there are often factors which have been shown to moderate the effects and delay onset. We will begin with a review of some established *risk factors*, which increase the likelihood of developing dementia, and then consider how some of these effects can be offset by *protective factors*, which reduce the likelihood.

Dementia and Age: An Accumulation of Events

It is generally considered that age is the biggest risk factor for developing dementia. However, this can be overstated in a way which implies that dementia is solely a disease of later life, which not the case. Whilst it is true that the prevalence of the most common forms of dementia (e.g. Alzheimer's and vascular dementia) increases with age, this does not apply to every dementia type. In fact, Alzheimer's disease was originally thought of as early-onset dementia, and the original patient documented by Alois Alzheimer (1907) was only 51 years old when he encountered her. Table 1.3 shows the average age of onset for several different forms of dementing disorders.

Kelley et al. (2008) looked at causes of dementia in a sample of 235 patients aged 17–45, and reported that degenerative disorders were the most common cause in those aged 35–45, whereas dementia in patients aged 17–35 was mainly attributable to other causes (e.g. metabolic or autoimmune disorders). Although degenerative disorders were rare under the age of 29, their youngest patient with FTD was aged 20. Only four cases of Alzheimer's disease were seen in this age range (2%), which contrasts with studies looking at a later age of onset. For example, Harvey et al. (2003) reported that in a group of patients with dementia below the age of 65, Alzheimer's disease accounted for 34% of diagnoses.

It is important to note that whilst some cultures have traditionally regarded dementia as a normal part of the ageing process, this is not the view currently held within the scientific community. There are a number of risk factors for dementia (described in the following

Table 1.3 Examples of average age of onset for different dementia types

Disorder	Typical age of onset
Alzheimer's disease, late onset	65+. Prevalence increases with age (Alzheimer's Society, 2020a)
Vascular dementia	65+. Risk of developing vascular dementia doubles every five years over the age of 65 (Alzheimer's Society, 2020b)
Dementia with Lewy bodies	50–70 (Schoenberg & Duff, 2011)
Frontotemporal dementia (FTD)	49–61 (Moore et al., 2020)
CADASIL (a rare genetic form of vascular dementia)	30–50 (Alzheimer's Society, 2020c)
Huntington's disease	30–40 (Keum et al., 2016)
Lysosomal storage diseases	Infancy to early adult (Platt et al., 2018)

sections) which increase with age. It is also known that a number of cognitive changes occur as part of the 'normal' ageing process, with a general slowing of the speed of cognitive processing being thought to underlie many changes in other domains (Salthouse, 2010). There is divided opinion regarding how to view the ageing process, with research in the area growing. Some researchers advocate that ageing itself should be viewed as a disease (e.g. Sinclair, 2019), whereas others state that 'ageing is not pathological' (Jamadar, 2019, p. 21). However, the thing to consider is that as we age, we lose brain cells which are not replaced. The state of a person's brain at any given time point represents the accumulation of events which have resulted in cell loss, and the older you are the more of those events you will have experienced. However, the speed at which different events occur, or different toxic agents accumulate, can vary greatly depending on the presence or absence of different *risk factors* which are likely to speed things up. There are also *protective factors* which either slow things down or act as a buffer against toxic effects.

Another reason why dementia increases with age is that the accumulation of toxic agents can progress very slowly, going largely unnoticed until the ensuing loss of brain cells reaches a critical level, below which the effect on cognitive abilities becomes more apparent. For example, there is evidence the protein abnormalities seen in Alzheimer's disease can start to accumulate whilst individuals are in their twenties, even though the effects may not become apparent until they are in their seventies (Braaks & Braaks, 1997). It has been suggested that rather than interpreting dementia as a disease of old age, it may be more realistic to view it as something which develops so slowly that it can take five decades or more before the effects become apparent (Braaks et al., 2011).

Genetics and Epigenetics

Sometimes dementia runs in families, with 25% of people aged over 55 having a first-degree relative affected (Slooter et al., 1998). Early-onset forms of dementia are more commonly associated with a genetic link (Sampson, Warren, & Rosner, 2004; Seshadri, Drachman, & Lippa, 1995). Although several members of a family having dementia increases the likelihood of a genetic link, it is important to remember that they will often have shared the same environment and customs. For instance, Kuru is a form of fatal neurodegenerative disorder which ran in families of the Fore people in Papua New Guinea. The presence of an abnormal protein, in this case a prion, was indeed central to the development of this disorder, but the mechanism by which it passed between generations was not genetic. Kuru was in fact an *infectious* disease, which was passed on via the funeral practices in the Fore culture, which included eating the dead (Mathews, Glasse, & Lindenbaum, 1968).

In the majority of *familial* cases, however, the common risk factor is likely to be genetic, which can take one of two forms: (1) a Mendelian type, which is caused by mutation in a single gene, or (2) a complex type, where genetics are a contributing factor (Loy et al., 2014). Genes underlying Mendelian forms of dementia are autosomal dominant, which means you can inherit the gene from one parent, as opposed to recessive genes which must be inherited from both parents. If you inherit one of these genes, there is a 95% chance of developing dementia (Loy et al., 2014). Examples of such genes include the amyloid precursor protein (APP), presenilin-1 (PSEN1), and presenilin-2 (PSEN2), which are related to roughly 5–10% of cases of early-onset Alzheimer's disease (Cacace, Sleegers, & Van Broeckhoven, 2016).

Loy et al. (2014) defined a complex disease model as one where normal variation in more than one gene interacts with environmental factors to increase the risk of developing dementia. The most well-known example is the APOE-E gene (Saunders et al., 1993), which has the strongest genetic link with late-onset Alzheimer's disease. There are three variants of this gene, one of which (ϵ4) increases the likelihood of developing Alzheimer's disease. According to the Alzheimer's Society, approximately 25% of the population have one copy of APOE-ϵ4, which doubles the risk of developing Alzheimer's disease. Roughly 2% of the population inherit this gene from both parents, which results in them being up to five times more likely to develop the disease (Alzheimer's Society, 2020d). It should be noted that not everyone with APOE-ϵ4 will develop dementia, and most cases of Alzheimer's disease occur sporadically without an *identified* genetic cause.

There are also hereditary, non-Alzheimer's forms of dementia, such as Huntington's disease and CADASIL. The latter is a rare autosomal-dominant disorder of the blood vessels, which leads to stroke and dementia with an average age of onset of 45 (Herfve & Chabriat, 2010).

Even in the case of dementias with a Mendelian pattern of inheritance, there is still evidence that protective factors can delay onset. Let us take the example of Huntington's disease (HD), which is a degenerative disorder associated with an abnormality in the huntingtin (HTT) gene that results in an overproduction of the protein huntingtin (McDonald et al., 1993), and is characterised by cognitive, motor, and psychiatric problems. There is currently no disease-modifying treatment nor means of delaying the onset of the disorder (Ho, 2019). The age of onset is determined by the number of times a particular series of three DNA building blocks (CAG) is repeated in the huntingtin gene (Trottier, Biancalana, & Mandel, 1994). However, in a retrospective study looking at the effects of lifestyle factors in HD patients, Trembath et al. (2010) found a difference of 4.6 years in age of onset between the most and the least active of their patients, taking into account the number of CAG repeats. There are also several mouse models of HD which suggest that an enriched environment may delay onset of HD symptoms, although this has yet to be demonstrated in clinical trials (Mees et al., 2019).

Blood Supply

As the health of any organ in the body is dependent upon a sufficient blood supply, it is unsurprising that risk factors for cardiovascular disease are also risk factors for stroke and dementia. If the blood supply to the brain is compromised, this will result in the death of brain cells. For example, memory deficits are often reported following cardiac arrests (Moulaert et al., 2009), which results in a lack of blood supply to the whole brain. When there is a sudden blockage of a major artery in the brain, damage ensues in the areas supplied by that blood vessel, which is known as an ischaemic stroke. This is usually characterised by a sudden onset, and a relatively focal area of damage caused by lack of oxygen and glucose, with accompanying inflammation (Lakhan et al., 2009). However, a loss of blood supply can also result from the progressive blockage of smaller blood vessels distributed in different regions, resulting in a more diffuse pattern of lesions and an accompanying decline in cognitive ability. Cognitive decline caused by cerebrovascular disease is referred to as vascular cognitive impairment (Dichgans & Leys, 2017).

Inflammation

There has been a great deal of interest in the role of chronic/long-term inflammation, both in the development of dementia and as a contributory factor to normal ageing (Woods et al., 2012). Whilst it is clear that inflammation occurs with ageing, and alongside many chronic health conditions, there remains some debate over whether it is a cause or a feature of dementia (Enciu & Popescu, 2013). Attempts to treat degenerative disorders using anti-inflammatory agents have yet to prove successful (Mason, Holmes, & Edwards, 2019).

Sleep and the Glymphatic System

Rather like inflammation, the effects of poor sleep have been a major feature of research over the last two decades. Sleep disturbance accompanies many chronic health problems, and there is often a question of whether this is a cause or an effect of the illness (Walker, 2018). The current consensus has moved towards a bidirectional relationship between poor sleep and dementia, with mechanisms put forward to explain how poor sleep contributes to the development of dementia, and how degeneration of certain brain areas leads to a reduced ability to sleep (Vaou et al., 2018).

The glymphatic system was first described by neuroscientist Maiken Nedergaard (Iliff et al., 2012), and in subsequent papers including Mestre, Mori, and Nedergaard (2020). Throughout the body, the lymphatic system operates for the removal of cellular waste. This system does not appear to be present within the brain, which has its own mechanism for waste removal: the glymphatic system. Glial cells within the brain carry out a similar function to the lymphatic system, and remove waste including toxic proteins such as beta amyloid and tau. The relationship with sleep arises because this system appears to predominantly operate during sleep and shows very little activity during wakefulness. Consequently, in degenerative disorders such as Alzheimer's and Parkinson's disease, which are associated with reduced quantity and quality of sleep, this system has less time to operate, making it less effective at clearing such proteins away.

Cognitive Reserve and Thresholds for Dementia

As mentioned earlier, one reason why the incidence of dementia increases with age is that many dementias take decades to develop. One explanation for why a degenerative disorder can develop without any clinical signs is that, throughout much of our lives, we have more brain cells than we need. We are born with all of our brain cells, and as part of maturation a pruning process takes place during which neural pathways, or circuits, are developed. As we age, we continue to lose brain cells, but we can function because we start off with more than we need. If the number of brain cells falls below a critical threshold level, problems with cognitive function become apparent, but if it remains above that level, the individual may continue to function as normal. For example, Katzman et al. (1989) described 10 cases of people who were found to have advanced Alzheimer's disease at post-mortem examination yet had shown no evidence of dementia whilst alive. All were found to have higher-than-average brain weights, and therefore more brain cells. This is known as neuronal, or cognitive, reserve (Stern, 2002).

Whilst the level of cognitive reserve an individual has may be difficult to measure directly, some attempt has been made to develop a cognitive reserve index based upon correlates such as years of education, occupation, and leisure activities (Nucci et al., 2012). In a longitudinal study of 12,280 participants aged over 50, Almeida-Meza, Steptoe, and Cadar (2021) found that those with higher levels of education, complex occupations, and multi-faceted leisure activities were less likely to develop dementia.

Connectomics

Another question which arises with different forms of dementia is why the presentations in a focal area have widespread consequences? This can partly be explained by the way the brain is organised, the understanding of which has changed greatly in recent years. From the nineteenth century onwards, there were debates about whether the brain is comprised of separate units, with different brain regions carrying out different functions, or whether functions were distributed throughout different regions. The current view can be seen as a meeting of these two apparently contradictory interpretations, with different areas designated to carry out specific processes as part of a circuit which incorporates other brain regions working together in an integrated fashion. So, a degenerative process concentrated in a specific area can have more widespread effects on cognitive function. For a review of connectomics, see Fornito et al. (2015). A change in the connectivity of these circuits, or networks, is seen as part of normal ageing. Older adults have lower connectivity within networks and higher connectivity between networks. This is illustrated in functional imaging studies of younger and older adults carrying out tasks, which show that older adults have less activity in task-relevant regions of the brain and more activity in non-task-relevant areas (Jamadar, 2019).

How Important Is Differential Diagnosis?

Even though there are currently no disease-modifying treatments available for most dementias, there are a number of reasons why knowing the most likely form of dementia is important. A part from differences in the use of current medication aimed at symptom relief, the progression of different diseases varies drastically in both time course and presentation. Whilst current technology only allows for a definitive diagnosis post-mortem, there has been an accumulation of data in recent decades which allows for probable diagnosis with a relatively high degree of certainty based upon the clinical presentation. Although some recent technological advances are leading to increasingly accurate diagnosis of some of the common disorders such as Alzheimer's disease, the most important information is still the clinical presentation, including, in many cases, the neuropsychological assessment.

The Role of Imaging and Biomarkers

Imaging has always been a central part of the diagnostic process, incorporating both CT and MRI scans. There have been some more recent developments, referred to as metabolic tests, which show potential for greatly increasing diagnosis accuracy. These include assessing cerebrospinal fluid for beta amyloid protein and looking at the distribution of beta amyloid protein via amyloid PET scans. Although these will be considered in more detail in subsequent chapters (e.g. Chapter 13), these techniques are mainly restricted to research settings and are not generally available in clinical practice.

The Scope of This Book

Many of the areas introduced here will be considered in more detail in subsequent chapters of this book which will consider in detail the diagnostic process, individual presentations, and development of interventions and preventative measures.

Key Points

- Dementia is a syndrome characterised by a progressive decline in cognitive abilities from a previous level, which is greater than would be expected with normal ageing and impacts upon day-to-day function.

- An acquired brain injury can also cause a decline in cognitive function, but is not a form of dementia as it is not progressive.

- Dementia affects roughly 7% of the population over the age of 65, and the World Health Organization lists it as the seventh most common cause of death.

- There are many diseases which can lead to dementia. Alzheimer's disease is the most common, accounting for up to 70% of cases.

- As a definitive diagnosis is currently only possible post-mortem, a probable diagnosis is made by considering converging information about the clinical presentation from different sources.

- Most forms of dementia are associated with the presence of a toxic agent, usually an abnormal form of protein which accumulates and causes cell death.

- Although there are some forms of rapid-onset dementia, most cases develop slowly over the course of years and decades before a significant decline in cognitive ability is seen.

- One reason why there are different forms of dementia is that different proteins are implicated, and the distribution of abnormal protein differs within the brain.

- "Available in routine clinical practice" Best put this in as some would claim recent trials on monoclonal antibody therapy drugs have been proven to be effective.

- There are currently no proven pharmacological treatments which slow down or stop the progression of dementia (disease-modifying), but there is evidence to suggest that lifestyle changes may achieve this to some extent.

- Research into dementia is ongoing, with the aim of developing pharmacological treatments which are truly disease-modifying.

References

Almeida-Meza, P., Steptoe, A., & Cadar, D. (2021). Is engagement in intellectual and social leisure activities protective against dementia risk? Evidence from the English Longitudinal Study of Ageing. *Journal of Alzheimer's Disease*, **80**(2), 555–65.

Alzheimer, A. (1907). Uber eine eigenaritage, schweren Erkrankung der Hirnrinde. *Allgemeine Zeitschrift für Psychiatrie und phychish-Gerichtliche Medizin (Berlin)*, **25**, 1134.

Alzheimer's Disease International. (2015). World Alzheimer Report 2015: The Global Impact of Dementia. www.alz.co.uk/researc h/WorldAlzheimerReport2015.pdf.

Alzheimer's Society (2020a). Risk factors for Alzheimer's disease. www.alzheimers.org.uk/ about-dementia/types-dementia/who-gets-al zheimers-disease#content-start

Alzheimer's Society (2020b). Who gets vascular dementia. www.alzheimers.org.uk/about-de

mentia/types-dementia/risk-factors-vascu
lar-dementia

Alzheimer's Society (2020c). What causes young onset dementia? https://bit.ly/3SdEkAJ.

Alzheimer's Society (2020d). Can genes cause dementia? www.alzheimers.org.uk/about-de mentia/risk-factors-and-prevention/alzhei mers-disease-and-genes

American Psychiatric Association (2000). *Diagnostic and Statistical Manual of Mental Disorders*, 4th ed. Washington, DC: American Psychiatric Association.

American Psychiatric Association (2013). *Diagnostic and Statistical Manual of Mental Disorders*, 5th ed. Washington, DC: American Psychiatric Association.

Avila, J., Santa-María, I., Pérez, M., Hernández, F., & Moreno, F. (2006). Tau phosphorylation, aggregation, and cell toxicity. *Journal of Biomedicine & Biotechnology*, **2006**(3), 74539. https://doi.or g/10.1155%2FJBB%2F2006%2F74539.

Bates, M. E., Bowden, S. C., & Barry, D. (2002). Neurocognitive impairment associated with alcohol use disorders: Implications for treatment. *Experimental and Clinical Psychopharmacology*, **10**(3), 193–212.

Bessen, R. A., & Marsh, R. F. (1992). Biochemical and physical properties of the prion protein from two strains of the transmissible mink encephalopathy agent. *Journal of Virology*, **66**, 2096–101.

Binder, L. I., Frankfurter, A., & Rebhun, L. I. (1985). The distribution of tau in the mammalian central nervous system. *Journal of Cell Biology*, **101**(4), 1371–8.

Braak, H., & Braak, E. (1997). Frequency of stages of Alzheimer-related lesions in different age categories. *Neurobiology of Aging*, **18**(4), 351–7.

Braak, H., Thal, D. R., Ghebremedhin, E., & Del Tredici, K. (2011). Stages of the pathologic process in Alzheimer disease: Age categories from 1 to 100 years. *Journal of Neuropathology & Experimental Neurology*, **70**(11), 960–9.

Cacace, R., Sleegers, K., & Van Broeckhoven, C. (2016). Molecular genetics of early-onset Alzheimer's disease revisited. *Alzheimer's & Dementia*, **12**(6), 733–48.

Cervós-Navarro, J., & Schumacher, K. (1994). Neurofibrillary pathology in progressive supranuclear palsy (PSP). *Journal of Neural Transmission*, Suppl; **42**, 153–64.

Chen, H., Epstein, J., & Stern, E. (2010). Neural plasticity after acquired brain injury: Evidence from functional neuroimaging. *Physical Medicine and Rehabilitation*, 2(125), S306–S312.

Collinge, J., Beck, J., Campbell, T., Estibeiro, K., & Will, R. G. (1996a) Prion protein gene analysis in new variant cases of Creutzfeldt–Jakob disease. *Lancet*, **348**, 56.

Day, E., Bentham, P., Callaghan, R., Kuruvilla, T., & George, S. (2004). Thiamine for Wernicke-Korsakoff syndrome in people at risk from alcohol abuse. *Cochrane Database of Systematic Reviews* (1).

de Silva, R., Lashley, T., Strand, C., et al. (2006). An immunohistochemical study of cases of sporadic and inherited frontotemporal lobar degeneration using 3R- and 4R-specific tau monoclonal antibodies. *Acta Neuropathologica*, **111**, 329–40.

Deary, I. J., Corley, J., Gow, A. J., et al. (2009). Age-associated cognitive decline. *British Medical Bulletin*, **92**, 135–52.

Delacourte, A. (2001). The molecular parameters of tau pathology: Tau as a killer and a witness. In M. Tolnay & A. Probst (Eds.), *Neuropathology and the Genetics of Dementia* (pp. 5–19). New York: Kluwer Academic/Plenum Publishers.

Delacourte, A., Sergeant, N., Wattez, A., et al. (1998) Vulnerable neuronal subsets in Alzheimer's and Pick's disease are distinguished by their tau isoform distribution and phosphorylation. *Annals of Neurology*, **43**, 193–204.

Dichgans, M., & Leys, D. (2017). Vascular cognitive impairment. *Circulation Research*, **120**, 573–91.

Enciu, A.-M., & Popescu, B. (2013). Is there a causal link between inflammation and dementia? *Biomedical Research International*, **2013**, Article ID 316495.

Fornito, A., Zalesky, A., & Breakspeare, M. (2015). The connectomics of brain disorders. *Nature Reviews: Neuroscience*, **16**, 159–72.

Fox, N. (2019). Imaging in dementia. *Journal of Neurological Sciences*, **405** (supplement), 16–17.

Gibb, W. R. G., Esiri, M. M., & Lees, A. J. (1987). Clinical and pathological features of diffuse cortical Lewy body disease (Lewy body dementia). *Brain*, **110**, 1131–53.

Giraud, T. D., Thompson, J. L., Pandharipande, P. P., et al. (2018). Clinical phenotypes of delirium during critical illness and severity of subsequent long-term cognitive impairment: A prospective cohort study. *The Lancet*, **6**(3), 213–22.

Glenner, C. C., & Wong, C. W. (1984). Alzheimer's disease: Initial report of the purification and characterization of a novel cerebrovascular amyloid protein. *Biochemistry and Biophysical Research Communications*, **120**, 885–90.

Goldman, M. S. (1983). Cognitive impairment in chronic alcoholics: Some cause for optimism. *American Psychologist*, **38**(10), 1045–54.

Harvey, R. J., Skelton-Robinson, M., & Rossor, M. N. (2003). The prevalence and causes of dementia in people under the age of 65 years. *Journal of Neurology, Neurosurgery and Psychiatry*, **74**, 1206–9.

Hervé, D., & Chabriat, H. (2010). CADASIL. *Journal of Geriatric Psychiatry and Neurology*, **23**(4), 269–76.

Ho, A. K. (2019). Huntington's disease. In D. R. Hocking, J. L. Bradshaw, & J. Fielding (Eds.), *Degenerative Disorders of the Brain* (pp. 88–155). Oxford: Routledge.

Iliff, J. J., Wang, M., Liao, Y., et al. (2012). A paravascular pathway facilitates CSF flow through the brain parenchyma and the clearance of interstitial solutes, including amyloid β. *Science Translational Medicine*, **4**(147), 147ra111. https://doi.org/10.1126/scitranslmed.3003748.

Jamadar, S. (2019). Brain circuitry in ageing and neurodegenerative disease. In D. R. Hocking, J. L. Bradshaw and J. Fielding (Eds.), *Degenerative Disorders of the Brain* (pp. 1–31). New York: Routledge.

Jessen, N. A., Munk, A. S. F., Lundgaard, I., & Nedergaard, M. (2015). The glymphatic system: A beginner's guide. *Neurochemical Research*, **40**, 2583–99.

Kalish, V. B., Gillham, J. E., & Unwin, B. K. (2014). Delirium in older persons: Evaluation and management. *American Family Physician*, **90**(3), 150–8.

Kanaan, N. M., Himmelstein, D. S., Ward, S. M., Combs, B., & Binder, L. I. (2015). Tau protein: Biology and pathobiology. In M. S. LeDoux (Ed.), *Movement Disorders: Genetics and Models*, 2nd ed. (pp. 857–74). London: Academic Press.

Katzman, R., Aronson, M., & Fuld, P., et al. (1989). Development of dementing illnesses in an 80-year-old volunteer cohort. *Annals of Neurology*, **25**, 317–324.

Kelley, B. J., Boeve, B. F., & Josephs, K. A. (2008). Young-onset dementia: Demographic and etiologic characteristics of 235 patients. *Archives of Neurology*, **65**, 1502–8.

Keum, J. W., Shin, A., Gillis, T., et al. (2016). The HTT CAG-expansion mutation determines age at death but not disease duration in Huntington disease. *American Journal of Human Genetics*, **98**(2), 287–98.

Kukreja, D., Günther, U., & Popp, J. (2015). Delirium in the elderly: Current problems with increasing geriatric age. *Indian Journal of Medical Research*, **142**(6), 655–62.

Laforce, R., Jr., Soucy, J. P., Sellami, L., et al. (2018). Molecular imaging in dementia: Past, present and future. *Alzheimer's and Dementia*, **14**(11), 1522–52.

Lakhan, S. E., Kirchgessner, A., & Hofer, M. (2009). Inflammatory mechanisms in ischemic stroke: Therapeutic approaches. *Journal of Translational Medicine*, **7**, 97.

Lim, A., Tsuang, D., Kukull, W., et al. (1999). Cliniconeuropathological correlation of Alzheimer's disease in a community-based case series. *Journal of the American Geriatric Society*, **47**, 564–9.

Loy, C. T., Schofield, P. R., Turner, A., & Kwok, J. B. J. (2014). The genetics of dementia. *Lancet*, **383**, 828–40.

MacDonald, M. E., Ambrose, C. M., Duyao, M. P., et al. (1993). A novel gene containing a trinucleotide repeat that is expanded and unstable on Huntington's disease chromosomes. *Cell*, **72**(6), 971–83.

MacQueen, G. M., & Memedovich, K. A. (2016). Cognitive dysfunction in major depression and bipolar disorder: Assessment and treatment. *Psychiatry and Clinical Neurosciences*, **71**(1), 18–27.

Mason, A., Holmes, C., & Edwards, C. (2019). Inflammation and dementia: Using rheumatoid arthritis as a model to develop treatments? *Autoimmunity Reviews*, **17**(9), 919–25.

Mathews, J. D., Glasse, R., & Lindenbaum, S. (1968). Kuru and cannibalism. *The Lancet*, **292**, 449–52.

Matthews, F. E., Stephan, B. C. M., Robinson, L., et al. (2016). A two-decade dementia incidence comparison from the cognitive function and ageing studies I & II. *Lancet*, **382**, 1405–12. https://doi.org/10.1038/ncomms11398.

McDermott, L. M., & Ebmeier, K. P. (2009). A meta-analysis of depression severity and cognitive function. *Journal of Affective Disorders*, **119**(1), 1–8.

McKhann, G., Drachman, D., Folstein, M., et al. (1984). Clinical diagnosis of Alzheimer's disease: report of the NINCDS-ADRDA Work Group under the auspices of Department of Health and Human Services Task Force on Alzheimer's Disease. *Neurology*, **34**, 939–44.

McKhann, G. M., Knopman, D. S., Chertkow, H., et al. (2011). The diagnosis of dementia due to Alzheimer's disease: Recommendations from the National Institute on Aging-Alzheimer's Association Workgroups on Diagnostic Guidelines for Alzheimer's Disease. *Alzheimer's & Dementia*, **7**, 263–9.

Mees, I., Tran, H., Renoir, T., & Hannan, A. J. (2019). Experience-dependent modulation of neurodegenerative disorders: Huntington's disease as an exemplar. In D. R. Hocking, J. L. Bradshaw & J. Fielding (Eds.), *Degenerative Disorders of the Brain*. Oxford: Routledge.

Mestre, H., Mori, Y., & Nedergaard, M. (2020). The brain's glymphatic system: Current controversies. *Trends in Neurosciences*, **43**(7), 458–66.

Moore, K. M., Nicholas, J., Grossman, M., et al. (2020). Age at symptom onset and death and disease duration in genetic frontotemporal dementia: An international retrospective cohort study. *Lancet Neurology*, **19**(2), 145–56.

Moulaert, V. R., Verbunt J. A., van Heugten, C. M., Wade, D. T. (2009). Cognitive impairments in survivors of out-of-hospital cardiac arrest: A systematic review. *Resuscitation*, **80**(3), 297–305.

Neumann, M., Sampathu, D. M., Kwong, L. K., et al. (2006). Ubiquitinated TDP-43 in frontotemporal lobar degeneration and amyotrophic lateral sclerosis. *Science*, **314**(5796), 130–3.

NHS Digital. (2020). Recorded Dementia Diagnoses – March 2020. https://digital.nhs.uk/data-and-information/publications/statistical/recorded-dementia-diagnoses/march-2020.

Nolan, M., Talbot, K., & Ansorge, O. (2016). Pathogenesis of FUS-associated ALS and FTD: insights from rodent models. *Acta Neuropathologica Communications*, **4**, 99. https://doi.org/10.1186/s40478-016-0358-8.

Nucci, M., Mapelli, D., & Mondini, S. (2012). Cognitive Reserve Index questionnaire (CRIq): A new instrument for measuring cognitive reserve. *Ageing Clinical and Experimental Research*, **24**(3), 218–26.

Nudo, R. J. (2011). Neural basis of recovery after brain injury. *Journal of Communication Disorders*, **44**(5), 515–20.

Petersen, R. C. (2016). Mild cognitive impairment. *Dementia*, **22**(2), 404–18.

Petersen, R. C., Smith, G. E., Waring, S. C., et al. (1999). Mild cognitive impairment: Clinical characterisation and outcome. *Archives of Neurology*, **56**(3), 303–8.

Platt, F. M., d'Azzo, A., Davidson, B. L., et al. (2018). Lysosomal storage diseases. *Nature Reviews Disease Primers*, **4**, 27.

Prince, M. et al. (2014). Dementia UK: Update Second Edition report produced by King's College London and the London School of Economics for the Alzheimer's Society. www.alzheimers.org.uk/sites/default/files/migrate/downloads/dementia_uk_update.pdf.

Ridley, N. J., Draper, B., & Withall, A. (2013). Alcohol-related dementia: An update of the evidence. *Alzheimers Research and Therapy*, **5**(1), 3.

Rosso, S. M., Kamphorst, W., de Graaf, B., et al. (2001). Familial frontotemporal dementia with ubiquitin-positive inclusions is linked to chromosome 17q21–2. *Brain*, **124**(Pt 10), 1948–57.

Roy, R., Niccolini, F., Pagano, G., et al. (2016). Cholinergic imaging in dementia spectrum disorders. *European Journal of Nuclear Medicine & Molecular Imaging*, **43**, 1376–86.

Sachdeva, A., Chandra, M., Choudhary, M., Dayal, P., & Anand, K. S. (2016). Alcohol-related dementia and neurocognitive impairment: A review study. *International Journal of High Risk Behaviors & Addiction*, **5**(3), e27976.

Salthouse, T. (2010). Selective review of cognitive ageing. *Journal of the International Neuropsychological Society*, **16**, 754–60.

Sampson, E. L., Warren, J. D., & Rossor, M. N. (2004). Young onset dementia. *Postgraduate Medical Journal*, **80**, 125–39.

Saunders, A. M., Blennow, K., Breteler, M. M. B., et al. (1993). Association of apolipoprotein E allele ε4 with late-onset familial and sporadic Alzheimer's disease. *Neurology*, **43**(8), 1467.

Schneider, J. A., Arvanitakis, Z., Bang, W., & Bennett, D. A. 2007. Mixed brain pathologies account for most dementia cases in community-dwelling older persons. *Neurology*, **69**(24), 2197–204.

Schoenberg, M. R., & Duff, K. (2011). Dementias and mild cognitive impairment in adults. In M. R. Schoenberg & J. G. Scott (Eds.), *The Little Black Book of Neuropsychology*. New York: Springer.

Selkoe, D., & Hardy, J. (2016). The amyloid hypothesis of Alzheimer's disease at 25 years. *EMBO Molecular Medicine*, **8**(6), 595–608.

Seshadri, S., Drachman, D. A., & Lippa, C. F. (1995). Apolipoprotein E epsilon 4 allele and the lifetime risk of Alzheimer's disease: What physicians know, and what they should know. *Archives of Neurology*, **52**, 1074–9.

Sinclair, D. A., & LaPlante, M. D. (2019). *Lifespan: Why We Age – And Why We Don't Have To*. New York: Atria Books.

Slooter, A. J., Cruts, M., Kalmijn, S., et al. (1998). Risk estimates of dementia by apolipoprotein E genotypes from a population-based incidence study: The Rotterdam Study. *Archives of Neurology*, **55**(7), 964–8.

Spillantini, M. G., Crowther, R. A., Jakes, R., et al. (1998). α-Synuclein in filamentous inclusions of Lewy bodies from Parkinson's disease and dementia with Lewy bodies. *Proceedings of the National Academy of Sciences of the United States of America*, **95**, 6469–73.

Stern, Y. (2002). What is cognitive reserve? Theory and research application of the reserve concept. *Journal of the International Neuropsychological Society*, **8**, 448–60.

Thomson, A. D., Cook, C. C., Touquet, R., & Henry, J. A. (2002). The Royal College of Physicians report on alcohol: Guidelines for managing Wernicke's encephalopathy in the accident and emergency. *Alcohol and Alcoholism*, **37**(6), 513–21.

Trembath, M. K., Horton, Z. A., Tippett, L., et al. (2010). A retrospective study on the impact of lifestyle on age at onset of Huntington's disease. *Movement Disorders*, **25**(10), 1444–50.

Trojanowski, J., Goedert, M., & Iwatsubo, T., et al. (1998). Fatal attractions: Abnormal protein aggregation and neuron death in Parkinson's disease and Lewy body dementia. *Cell Death & Differentiation*, **5**, 832–7.

Trottier, Y. V., Biancalana, J. L., & Mandel, J. (1994). Instability of CAG repeats in Huntingtons disease: Relation to parental transmission and age of onset. *Journal of Medical Genetics*, **31**(5), 377–82.

Vaou, O. E., Lin, S. H., Branson, C., et al. (2018). Sleep and dementia. *Current Sleep Medicine Reports*, **4**, 134–42.

Walker, M. (2018). *Why we sleep*. Penguin Books Limited.

Winblad, B., Palmer, K., Kivipelto, M., et al. (2004). Mild cognitive impairment – Beyond controversies, towards a consensus: Report of the International Working Group on Mild Cognitive Impairment. *Journal of Internal Medicine*, **256**, 240–6.

Woods, J. A., Wilund, K. R., Martin, S. A., & Kistler, B. (2012). Exercise, inflammation and aging. *Aging and Disease*, **3**(1), 130–40.

World Health Organization (2018). *International Classification of Diseases*, 11th edition.

Chapter 2

Diagnosing Dementia

Diagnosis and Formulation

There is currently no definitive test for dementia or its subtypes. A definitive diagnosis can only be confirmed post-mortem. Diagnosis therefore proceeds by accumulating evidence and arriving at a conclusion, eliminating other possibilities along the way. The word 'diagnosis' entered the English language during the seventeenth century, and usually means the art or act of identifying a disease from its signs and symptoms (Merriam-Webster, 2020). Formulation refers to the 'putting together of components in appropriate relationships or structures, according to a formula' (https://en.wikipedia .org/wiki/Formulation). In most instances, the diagnosis of dementia proceeds by a formulation process, with a 'probable' diagnosis being the end point. It is important to acknowledge that this is an imperfect process, as illustrated by Beach et al.'s (2012) report that expert diagnosis of Alzheimer's disease will still be wrong in 20% of cases. In this chapter, we will go through the process of information gathering which is required to arrive at a diagnosis of dementia.

Expert and Novice Diagnosticians

Psychologists have researched expert and novice differences for many decades, in many areas of decision-making, including medical diagnosis. Experts know more about their area of study, and are better at applying that knowledge (Kolodner, 1983). Experts also make more use of and have superior recall of contextual information (Hobus, Boshuizen, & Schmidt, 1990). Shubert et al. (2013) compared emergency doctors with one year of experience to those with many years of experience and reported five key differences (see Table 2.1).

Establishing a Context

The purpose of taking a history is to establish a context. The type of information required is that which is relevant to establishing this context, and includes risk factors for developing dementia and other factors which might impact upon cognitive function. A review of some of the risk factors was included in Chapter 1. Here we list some recommendations for the type of information to collect, along with the possible relevance. Table 2.2 lists examples. This list is not exhaustive, and in some cases there may be relevant information which is not included here. However, it is important not to take an overly extensive history which includes material of no relevance to the diagnosis.

Table 2.1 Differences between expert and novice emergency doctors, taken from Shubert et al. (2013)

Experts	Novices
More able to extract relevant information from a large body of data	Found extracting relevant information more difficult
Focussed more on the nature of the situation	Focussed more on possible courses of action
More willing to alter diagnostic direction in light of new information	Reluctant to accept new information which was not consistent with their diagnosis
Paid more attention to patient context	Paid more attention to objective data rather than context
Found it easier to incorporate information into the bigger picture	Found it more difficult to fit information into the bigger picture

Table 2.2 Suggested relevant information to collect when taking a clinical history to establish a context

Information	Possible relevance
Date of birth and age	The likelihood of developing different types of dementia changes with age. Different dementias are more common in certain age ranges
Educational and occupational background, including highest level of qualification attained	This information is helpful in establishing an estimate of premorbid ability
Current occupational status	This is relevant in establishing the person's current level of function, and whether it has declined (e.g. did they stop working as a result of cognitive difficulties)
Current level of everyday function, and kind of problems they are encountering	A decline in function is required for a diagnosis of dementia. The initial presenting symptoms can be an indicator of the type of dementia
Time course and pattern of onset	The period over which problems developed can be a crucial diagnostic factor. The pattern of onset can also point towards the underlying cause (e.g. steady and gradual, stepwise or fluctuating)
Medical history	A number of medical and chronic health conditions are associated with cognitive decline
History of stroke or acquired brain injury	Stoke and acquired brain injury are both associated with cognitive decline, and both carry an increased risk of developing dementia
Sensory problems (e.g. hearing and vision)	Sensory problems can impede someone's ability to complete a cognitive test. Hearing problems are also a risk factor for cognitive decline

Table 2.2 (cont.)

Information	Possible relevance
Hallucinations or delusions	These can be indicative of certain types of dementia, but also can indicate severe mental health problems
Vascular risk factors (e.g. high blood pressure, elevated cholesterol, diabetes, history of heart disease or atrial fibrillation)	These are risk factors for numerous forms of dementia, including vascular dementia
Quantity and quality of sleep	Poor sleep is associated with reduced cognitive function, and long-term sleep difficulties are a risk factor for dementia
Lifestyle factors such as smoking, alcohol consumption, poor diet, and lack of exercise	These are risk factors for developing dementia
Family history of dementia	A strong family history of dementia, particularly early onset, can be a risk factor
Family history of neurological problems, stroke, or other vascular issues	A strong family history can be a risk factor
Medication	Some medicines are sedating, and others have an anti-cholinergic burden. Both can affect cognitive function
Current or past mental health problems	These can impact upon cognitive function, and be risk factors for developing dementia

Establishing Whether Someone Has Dementia?

Working through the diagnostic process in stages is recommended:

Stage 1:

   A. Establish whether there is evidence for a decline in cognitive function

   B. Establish whether there is evidence for a decline in everyday function

Stage 2:

   A. Consider whether the evidence meets the criteria for dementia (i.e. a decline in two areas of cognition *and* a decline in everyday function)

   B. Consider whether the evidence meets the criteria for mild cognitive impairment (i.e. a decline in cognition, but relatively well-preserved everyday function). Identify if any factors other than the early stages of a progressive disorder might account for the presentation (e.g. depression, chronic health problems)

   C. If neither criterion is met, consider if there are any other factors which might account for the presenting difficulties

Stage 3:

   A. Having established the person meets the criteria for dementia, consider whether there may be other, potentially reversible, factors which could account for the presentation (e.g. delirium)

B. If other possible causes have been investigated/ruled out, proceed to evaluate the clinical presentation and other forms of investigations (e.g. scans, bloods, neuropsychology, biomarkers if available) to determine the most likely type of dementia

Evidence for Cognitive Impairment

Establishing whether someone has experienced an objective decline in cognitive function will always involve some form of cognitive testing. Although an individual's subjective impression of cognitive decline can be a predictor of future decline, it is not uncommon for people to experience a subjective decline whilst performing within the expected range on objective testing (Parfenov et al., 2020). In fact, placing too much emphasis on an individual's subjective appraisal of their memory can reduce diagnostic accuracy in cases of MCI (Lenehan, Klekociuk, & Summers, 2012).

In many cases, the presence of cognitive impairment may be determined using a screening instrument such as the Addenbrookes Cognitive Evaluation (ACE-III) (Hodges et al., 2017; Mathurinath et al., 2000) or the Montreal Cognitive Assessment (MoCA) (Nasreddine et al., 2005). Screening instruments use a cut-off score, which has been determined to give the best balance between sensitivity (the ability to correctly detect true cases) and specificity (the ability to correctly reject healthy patients). When deciding which tool is most appropriate for a particular service, consideration should be given to the context in which it is to be administered and the time available. A list of common screening instruments is given in Table 2.3.

To use a screening instrument correctly, it is necessary to know the cut-off score and the age range for which it is suitable. For instance, the ACE-III recommends using a cut-off score of 82/100 for maximum specificity, and 88/100 for maximum sensitivity. It is intended for use in individuals over the age of 50. There are three parallel versions intended for repeat/serial assessment. The MoCA uses a cut-off of 24/30 and has been validated for individuals aged 55–85. There are three forms of the MoCA, although there has been some suggestion that they are not strictly parallel (Siciliano et al., 2019). These instruments also give a cognitive profile, which can be informative in distinguishing different dementia types (Hsieh et al., 2013; Mathuranath et al., 2000).

Whilst screening instruments may be adequate for a large number of patients seen within a memory assessment service, there will be some patients for whom the results are not sufficiently clear, such as those with premorbid ability considerably above or below average. Whilst there have been suggestions of using different cut-off scores for such people, it is difficult to find agreement on exactly how to adjust the cut-off. In such instances a more extensive neuropsychology assessment is likely to be useful, which would include an estimate of premorbid ability to allow for a more reliable appraisal of whether there has been cognitive decline from premorbid ability levels. This book includes a chapter on the use of neuropsychological assessment in the diagnosis of dementia (see Chapter 4), but it is worth briefly considering some areas of confusion which sometimes arise in clinical practice.

1. A neuropsychological assessment is only appropriate when it is considered that there remains some ambiguity regarding whether a decline in function has occurred. If it is clear from the cognitive screen that there has been a significant deterioration, further testing is unlikely to be justified or informative.

Table 2.3 Examples of cognitive screening instruments in common use

Test	Brief comment
Mini-Mental State Examination (MMSE) (Folstein, Folstein & McHugh, 1975)	Thirty questions. Takes 5–10 minutes to administer. Previously free to use, and very popular. Now copyrighted and no longer free.
Mini Cog (Borson et al., 2000)	Three-word recall and clock drawing. Takes 5–10 minutes to administer. Free to use.
General Practitioner Assessment of Cognition (GPCOG). (Brodaty et al., 2002)	Patient-based test with informant questionnaire. Up to 10 minutes to administer both components. Free to use.
Six item cognitive impairment test (Katzman et al., 1983)	Six questions. Takes less than 5 minutes to administer. Free to use.
Montreal Cognitive Assessment (MoCA) (Nasreddine et al., 2005)	Thirty items; 10 minutes administration time. Widely used. Users are required to complete training, for which there is a fee. Shortened version MoCA-Blind also available, which can be administered by phone.
Addenbrookes Cognitive Examination (ACE) (Mathuranath et al., 2000)	Currently in third edition. Features four parallel versions for repeat testing; 19 items which assess 5 cognitive domains. Roughly 20 minutes to administer. Free to use. Online training available.
CANTAB Mobile (Barnett et al., 2015)	Features one test: visual paired associate learning. Administered via iPad; 10 minutes to administer. Not open use, and requires suitable device (iPad).

2. Neuropsychological testing is likely to be most informative in the early stages of cognitive decline. This is because a cognitive profile is based upon the pattern of strengths and weaknesses, which is most apparent in the early stages of a progressive disorder. As dementia becomes more advanced, most aspects of cognitive function become affected, which translates into a relatively flat pattern of global impairment. If all aspects of cognition are impaired, the neuropsychological assessment is unlikely to contribute much to differential diagnosis.

3. Following on from this, accurately applying criteria for MCI (e.g. Winblad et al., 2004) is likely to require more than a screening instrument.

4. If an individual has been relatively high functioning (e.g. extensive education and/or an occupation which is cognitively demanding), a neuropsychological assessment would be recommended as it may be possible for a considerable decline in function to have occurred but for the individual to remain above cut-off on a screening instrument. A neuropsychological assessment would hopefully be able to compare current cognitive function to an estimate of premorbid cognitive function. Conversely, if someone has less education, a cognitively undemanding occupation, or no occupation, a score below cut-off on a screening instrument may not indicate cognitive decline from a previous level.

5. Cognitive tests should not be done in isolation. One of the themes of this book in relation to assessment is the importance of context. It is not uncommon to receive

a referral request to assess somebody's memory or executive function, or their premorbid ability. A test of a specific aspect of cognitive function is only meaningful in the context of other tests with which to compare it. We are always looking for strengths and weaknesses, which cannot be determined if there are no other tests against which to compare.

Regarding how much of a decline is required for a diagnosis, DSM-V recommends a discrepancy of between one and two standard deviations below 'appropriate norms' for a diagnosis of minor neurocognitive disorder. The revised criteria for MCI (Albert et al., 2011) recommended '1 to 1.5 standard deviations below the mean for their age and education matched peers on culturally appropriate normative data' (p. 272). For major neurocognitive disorder (dementia), DSM-V recommends two or more standard deviations (American Psychiatric Association, 2013).

Establishing a Change in Everyday Function

The issue of whether someone has experienced a functional decline can lead to prolonged debate in multidisciplinary team meetings. Although a functional decline is considered essential for the diagnosis of dementia, there seems to be little consistency regarding how much of a decline is required, and how best to measure this. As with cognitive function, a person's premorbid ability should be taken into account wherever possible, as a high-functioning individual may experience a considerable decline yet still be able to carry out basic and instrumental activities of daily living (ADLs). Conversely, these abilities may be lost following a relatively small decline in someone functioning at the other end of the ability range.

DSM-V states that the cognitive decline in dementia should be sufficient to 'interfere with independence in everyday activities (i.e. at a minimum, requiring assistance with complex instrumental activities of daily living such as paying bills or managing medications)' (APA, 2013, p. 602). Albert et al. (2011) state that for a diagnosis of MCI the person may be less efficient and more error-prone, but they generally maintain independence with minimal aids or assistance. The distinction between MCI and dementia in terms of function therefore appears to be (1) if a person can still do everything, albeit with more effort, it is MCI; (2) if there are things they are no longer able to do, it is dementia.

There are three different approaches to assessing function: (1) self-report, (2) informant report, and (3) performance-based measures, where someone is observed carrying out certain tasks. Whilst performance-based assessments may appear to be the best approach, this is often time-consuming and is likely to require specialised training, and there may be restrictions on which professions are able to complete such assessments. As is the case with reports of cognitive ability, self-reports of performance may be unreliable, particularly if insight is lost, as is often found when dementia progresses (DeBettignies, Mahurin, & Pirozzolo, 1990). Consequently, informant-based reports are frequently used for this purpose as they will hopefully be based upon a rating from someone who knows the person well and they are relatively easy to administer. Unfortunately, a risk will always remain regarding how accurate the informant's rating may be. Table 2.4 lists several instruments which are commonly used to assess function. Some challenges to consider when choosing a suitable instrument are (1) many instruments assess only current function rather than change in function, (2) difficulties due to a change in mobility are often not clearly separated from difficulties due to a change in cognition, (3) instruments based on observer reports introduce a degree of subjectivity, and (4) the use of some instruments requires training or is limited to certain professions.

Table 2.4 Examples of instruments to assess function

Instrument	Comments
The Bristol Activities of Daily Living Scale (BADLS) (Bucks et al., 1996)	Twenty item questionnaire to be completed by a carer, who rates the person's current proficiency in different areas.
Everyday Cognition Questionnaire (Ecog) (Farias et al., 2008), with a shortened version (Tomaszewski Farias et al., 2011)	Thirty-nine item informant questionnaire, with 12-item shortened version (ECog–12).
Functional Activities Questionnaire (Pfeffer et al., 1982)	Ten item informant questionnaire.
Informant Questionnaire on Cognitive Decline in the Elderly (IQCode) (Jorm, Scott, &. Jacomb, 1989); short form (Jorm, 1994)	Sixteen-item informant questionnaire. Instead of rating the current level of performance, informants rate the degree of change which has occurred over a 10-year period.
Assessment of Motor and Processing Skills (Fisher, 1994)	Observational assessment tool where the individual performs two tasks, which are scored on a four-point scale according to defined criteria. Distinguishes between motor and cognitive ability.

Dementia Severity

DSM-V recommends the following classifications for dementia severity:

- Mild: Difficulties with instrumental ADLs (e.g. using technology such as a mobile phone, housework/housekeeping, shopping, using transport, preparing food, managing medication, managing finances).
- Moderate: Difficulties with basic ADLs (e.g. feeding, dressing, personal hygiene, bathing, managing continence).
- Severe: Fully dependent.

A number of instruments have been developed for the purpose of staging in dementia, as well as some screening instruments being used for this purpose. For example, it has been suggested that a cut-off score of 61 on the ACE-III is useful for distinguishing mild from moderate dementia (Giebel and Challis, 2017). There are a number of dementia staging scales, with the Clinical Dementia Rating (CDR) being the best evidenced and also available in multiple languages (Rikkert et al., 2011). The CDR has some drawbacks in that it takes 30 minutes to administer, and some clinical judgement is required in administration and scoring (Moetler et al., 2015). The Dementia Severity Rating Scale (DSRS) is a 12-item informant-rating scale which may serve as a shorter alternative (Clark & Ewbank, 1996), and has good predictive value when compared to the CDR (Moetler et al., 2015). A limitation of such scales is that they tend to be quite Alzheimer-centric and may therefore be of less use in staging other forms of dementia.

Things to Consider Other Than Dementia

As dementia is not the only cause of cognitive decline, it is important to consider other possible contributing factors. This is either to rule them out as alternative explanations or to evaluate whether there may be additional factors which may be amenable to intervention. The following sections discuss some possible factors, but in no way constitute an exhaustive list.

Delirium

Although likely to be less of a problem in community settings, delirium is often seen in hospital settings, and has been reported in up to a third of patients in intensive care units (Salluh et al., 2015). It is defined as an acute, fluctuating syndrome of altered attention, awareness, and cognition (Kalish, Gillham, & Unwin, 2014), which may result from multiple factors but is usually reversible. Although delirium is not dementia, it may be mistaken for dementia, and can occur in patients with dementia, giving an exaggerated impression of dementia severity. It is associated with an underlying medical condition, such as an infection, and treatment proceeds by targeting the underlying illness.

Mental Health Problems

Mental health problems, particularly severe disorders such as psychosis and major depressive disorder, are known to impact upon cognitive ability. It is important to be aware of the presence of such problems, which can be identified by clinical interview and accessing patient notes. A mood inventory is also recommended, such as the Hospital Anxiety and Depression Scale (HADS) (Zigmond & Snaith, 1983), which is widely used in healthcare settings and has been shown to have some validity in patients with dementia (Scott et al., 2017).

Psychosis is associated with a range of cognitive disorders (Elvevag & Goldberg, 2000), to the extent that any cognitive assessment carried out during the course of a florid psychosis would be considered unreliable. There is evidence for improved cognitive function following the use of antipsychotic medication (Harvey & Keefe, 2001); however, the relationship is not straightforward as anti-psychotics can lead to metabolic problems, which in turn can have a negative effect on cognitive function (MacKenzie et al., 2018).

Medication

A number of different types of medication are associated with a decline in cognitive function. Although this is not an exhaustive list, the following are noteworthy:

- Anti-psychotics
- Anti-convulsants
- Anti-depressants
- Sedatives
- Pain relief
- Certain chemotherapy drugs
- Anti-cholinergics

A relationship between available levels of the neurotransmitter acetyl choline and cognitive function has been hypothesised for many years and underlies the rationale for many of the medications prescribed for Alzheimer's disease. Conversely, many medications are known to block acetyl choline receptors, which is known as anti-cholinergic burden (ACB). The extent to which this occurs with different types of drugs was first tabulated by Boustani et al. (2008), and can be looked up online via the ACB Calculator website created by Rebecca King and Steve Rabino (www.acbcalc.com/pages/about).

Sensory Impairment

Vision and hearing are the main senses used in a cognitive assessment or interview. It is important to ascertain whether a person has any sensory problems, and also if they have any aids to assist with this (e.g. glasses, hearing aid). Visual impairment has been associated with reduced cognitive test performance (Macnamara et al., 2021), although it is certainly possible to use non-visual screening instruments (e.g. MoCA-blind) and neuropsychological assessments can also be adapted to exclude visual items.

Hearing loss has also been associated with an increased risk of developing dementia (Lin et al., 2011; Liu & Lee, 2019). Lodeiro-Fernandez et al. (2015) looked at the effect of hearing loss on language test performance in healthy older adults and those with dementia. They concluded that hearing loss affected performance on comprehension tasks, but not on language production tasks (e.g. verbal fluency) in the non-dementia group. There was no relationship between hearing loss and performance on either form of test for the dementia group.

Medical Problems

Chronic health problems are also associated with cognitive decline. This has been reported in health problems such as chronic heart failure Vogels et al. (2007), respiratory disease (Antonelli Incalzi et al., 2003), rheumatoid arthritis (Shin et al., 2012), and chronic pain (Hart, Wade, & Martelli, 2003).

Although blood tests are not commonly used to identify different types of dementia, they are scrutinised to identify possibly reversible causes of cognitive impairment, such as infection, thyroid problems, vitamin deficiencies, and organ dysfunction. Though by no means an exhaustive list, Table 2.5 lists blood markers which may be considered.

Imaging

Dementia is diagnosed on the basis of objective tests of cognitive ability and reported or observational evaluation of everyday function. Whilst clinical presentation and cognitive profile can be indicative of the type of dementia, imaging technology is likely to play an increasingly important role in identifying the subtype. It should be noted that whilst imaging may be an important component, it cannot be the sole basis of diagnosis and a scan report stating 'no abnormality found' does not mean there is no disease present.

Structural imaging may be part of an evaluation, but the clinical assessment remains the primary method of determining whether a patient has dementia. Both CT and MRI imaging are used, with MRI traditionally having higher resolution which can be advantageous for identifying signs of ischaemic damage such as small vessel disease. However, a review and meta-analysis by Beynon et al. (2012) concluded that there was insufficient evidence to

Table 2.5 Examples of bio-markers which may be important when considering possible causes of cognitive decline

Urea and electrolytes	These are indicators of kidney function. Electrolyte disturbance can result in hyponatraemia. Hypercalcaemia can change mental state and create confusion
Glucose levels	Low blood-sugar levels (hypoglycaemia) can cause confusion
Vitamin B_{12} and folate (B_9)	Low levels are associated with cognitive impairment
C-reactive protein (CRP)	This is a protein produced by the liver. Elevated levels are an indication of inflammation, and levels are often raised at the start of an infection
Thyroid function tests (TFTs)	Hyperthyroidism is associated with anxiety and hyperactivity. Hypothyroidism is associated with depression, fatigue, and reduced cognitive function
Haemoglobin	Anaemia is associated with fatigue and reduced cognitive function
Liver blood tests, often referred to a liver function tests (LFTs)	These can be indicative of damage or inflammation of the liver. They include looking at the levels of alanine aminotransferase (ALT), aspartate aminotransferase (AST), alkaline phosphatase (ALP) and y-Glutamyltransferase (GGT), albumon, and bilirubin
Mid-steam urine sample	This can be an indicator of a urinary tract infection

conclude MRI was superior to CT for identifying cerebrovascular changes in autopsy-confirmed and clinical cohorts of VaD, AD, and 'mixed dementia'.

The three main purposes of structural imaging are:

1. To rule out other pathologies such as tumours.
2. To identify structural change due to volume loss, both overall (global) and if concentrated in a particular lobe or brain region.
3. To identify evidence of cerebrovascular disease such as white matter ischaemia and strategic infarcts.

Indicators of specific pathologies will be discussed in individual chapters. For a review of the use of structural imaging in dementia, see Harper et al. (2014).

Functional imaging techniques such as fMRI, Positron Emission Tomography (PET), and single-photon emission computed tomography (SPECT) focus on measuring changes in phyisiological variables rather than anatomy, such as metabolism, blood flow, chemical composition, and absorption. Their use is more common in research settings, although some have been introduced into clinical practice. For example, SPECT and PET can be used to demonstrate reduced dopamine uptake transporter (DaT) uptake in the basal ganglia, which can potentially distinguish Alzheimer's disease from dementia with Lewy bodies (McKeith et al., 2017). PET has greater specificity and sensitivity than SPECT but is usually less likely to be available in clinical practice (Bayer, 2018).

Molecular imaging such as amyloid PET scans and levels of beta amyloid and tau proteins in cerebral-spinal fluid (CSF) have featured prominently in the research literature.

These techniques have enormous potential to increase precision in diagnosing dementia subtypes, but as yet are not widely used in clinical practice.

Whilst imaging data can be useful, it is not always required and not always helpful. The NICE guideline on dementia (2018) recommends to 'offer structural imaging to rule out reversible causes of cognitive decline and to assist with subtype diagnosis, unless dementia is well-established and the subtype is clear'. The London Dementia Clinical Network (Orleans-Foley, Isaacs, & Cook, 2018) has published guidelines regarding when it may or may not be appropriate to request a scan as part of the process of dementia diagnosis.

Key Points

- Dementia is diagnosed on the basis of clinical presentation and function.
- There is no definitive test. Diagnosis proceeds by an accumulation of evidence, and a decision regarding a 'probable' diagnosis is made on the balance of probabilities.
- To arrive at a dementia diagnosis, there must be evidence of a decline in (1) cognitive ability and (2) everyday function from a previously higher level; (3) evidence of progression should also be present to distinguish from acquired brain injury.
- Consideration should be given to non-progressive and potentially reversible causes of decline, which should be ruled out before making a diagnosis of dementia.
- Unnecessary investigations should be avoided. However, when it is not possible to arrive at a conclusion on the basis of information presented, additional investigations such as neuropsychological assessments and specialist scans should be sought.

Appendix A   Case Studies

Case Study: LL

Presentation

LL is a 55-year-old female who was referred for assessment in relation to subjective cognitive problems which had been apparent since contracting COVID two years previously. She reported a further worsening of her cognition following a chest infection 18 months later. LL did not report a progression of symptoms since these incidents, and in fact felt there had been some improvement in recent weeks.

Her reported problems consisted of forgetting conversations, programmes she had watched on television, and recent events. She also reported word-finding problems, such as requesting 'second-hand stamps' at the post office instead of 'second class'. She noted that problems are more evident when she is tired, and she has experienced increased fatigue levels since contracting COVID.

Educational and Occupational Background

LL had left school at the age of 18 following A-levels. She then undertook degree-level training to become a healthcare professional. After several years working as a practitioner, she moved into management.

Activities of Daily Living

LL was still able to carry out both basic and instrumental ADLs (e.g. using technology, managing her finances, online shopping). She had been off work since contracting COVID, but recently commenced a phased return. At the time of the assessment, she was working three days a week, and reported the biggest challenge to be her levels of fatigue.

The IQcode was complete by her daughter with a score of 3.8, which is above the recommended cut-off of 3.31.

Cognitive Assessment

LL underwent screening with the ACE-III, on which her score was above the cut-off score. As this did not establish the presence of cognitive decline, she was referred to neuropsychology for further assessment. The results of this indicated that her immediate memory and attention scores were between 1 and 1.5 standard deviations lower than expected. Her delayed memory scores were between 1.5 and 2 standard deviations lower than expected. There was no evident decline in executive function.

Medical History

LL had no significant medical history prior to contracting COVID and experiencing a chest infection 18 months later. She had no vascular risk factors other than elevated cholesterol, which was corrected following prescription of statin medication.

She had recently started on a course of hormone replacement therapy, following which she reported some subjective improvement in her cognitive abilities. This and her statin were the only medications taken.

There was no significant history of mental health problems, although LL reported feeling stressed and anxious since contracting COVID.

Imaging Data

LL underwent an MRI scan, which was reported as showing no abnormalities.

Lifestyle Factors

LL had never consumed alcohol on a regular basis or used recreational drugs. She had smoked 10–20 cigarettes a day, but stopped altogether 25 years ago (age 30).

Family History

There was a family history of heart disease and late-onset dementia. Both of these tended to affect family members over the age of 70.

Blood Tests

Nothing was identified in her blood results to indicate infection or any form of organ dysfunction.

Conclusions

It was considered that LL had evidence of cognitive decline sufficient to meet the criteria for amnestic mild cognitive impairment. There was not clear evidence of a decline in function which could be clearly attributable to changes in her cognitive ability, and none of her cognitive scores were more than two standard deviations lower than expected: she therefore did not meet the criteria for dementia. The pattern of onset of two distinct periods of decline following episodes of physical illness, and reports of some recent improvement, did not fit the pattern of a progressive disorder. There was no evidence from her imaging data to indicate any abnormality.

It was considered most likely that any decline in cognitive function was related to her episodes of ill-health, and she remained under the care of the long-term COVID service.

Case Study: BS

Presentation

BS is a 75-year-old female who was referred for assessment in relation to subjective cognitive problems which had been developing gradually over a period of approximately five years. BS did not initially notice these herself, but found that her friends were pointing out that she repeated herself in conversation and frequently did not recall prior conversations. She reported good recall of distant events, but poor recall of recent events.

Reported problems in addition to forgetting conversations were leaving the oven on, forgetting appointments, and not keeping track of the plot of her favourite soap opera. She also reported occasional word-finding problems.

Educational and Occupational Background

BS had left school at the age of 15 without formal qualifications. She worked in retail, progressing to be an assistant manager of a medium-sized DIY shop. She retired at 60, and has since occupied herself by caravanning with her husband and attending a local church-run social group.

Activities of Daily Living

BS was still able to carry out basic ADLs but had passed on management of finances to her husband. She had previously used a computer, but now found this too difficult.

Cognitive Assessment

BS underwent screening with the MoCA, on which her score was considerably below the cut-off. Her weakest score was for memory items.

Medical History

BS had a history of high blood pressure and elevated cholesterol, both managed by medication. There had also been some significant weight gain since she retired. She described herself as 'never having been thin'.

She had experienced an episode of depression following the birth of her second child, although this responded to medication. There were no further episodes.

Imaging Data

BS underwent a CT scan, which reported 'global involutional changes', slightly more pronounced in the temporal lobes.

Lifestyle Factors

BS smoked 20 cigarettes a day until the age of 40. Her alcohol consumption had been limited to special occasions, and never exceeded two glasses of wine.

Family History

There was a family history of late-onset memory problems, although no formally diagnosed case of dementia.

Blood Tests

Blood test results did not indicate any signs of infection or any form of organ dysfunction.

Conclusions

It was considered that BS had evidence of cognitive decline and a change in function sufficient to meet the criteria for dementia. As she now required support to carry out some instrumental activities of daily living, but was fully independent with basic ADLs, this was diagnosed as mild dementia.

The onset had been gradual over several years. Her primary deficit on cognitive testing was in memory, and her CT scan report described atrophy more pronounced in the temporal lobes. The conclusion was that this was probable Alzheimer's disease.

Appendix B Dementia Checklist

History	Select appropriate option or supply information
Is the history suggestive of a decline in cognitive ability?	Yes/no
What is the age of the person?	• working age (under 65) • young old (65–74) • middle old (75–84) • oldest old (85+)
What was the pattern of onset?	• sudden • gradual • stepwise • fluctuating
What was the *initial* presenting sign/symptom?	
Cognition	
Is there evidence for a decline in cognitive function?	Yes/no/unsure
If unsure, refer for a neuropsychology assessment	Neuropsychology required? Yes/no
Everyday function	
Is there evidence for a change in function?	• no change • some change but can still do everything • help required with instrumental ADLs (e.g. use telephone, laundry and dressing, shopping and errands, transportation, meal preparation, medication management, housekeeping activities, managing finances).

(cont.)

History	Select appropriate option or supply information
	• help required w th basic ADLs (e.g. personal hygiene, dressing, eating/drinking, continence, transfers)
Other considerations	• medications wh ch could affect cognition
	• physical health problems
	• potentially reversible factors
	• possible functional explanations
Dementia or MCI?	• cognition and function → dementia
	• cognition, but not function → MCI
	• change in function but not cognition → consider other explanations (e.g. physical, functional)
	• no change in cognition, no change in function → no diagnosis

Appendix C MCI/Dementia Decision Tree

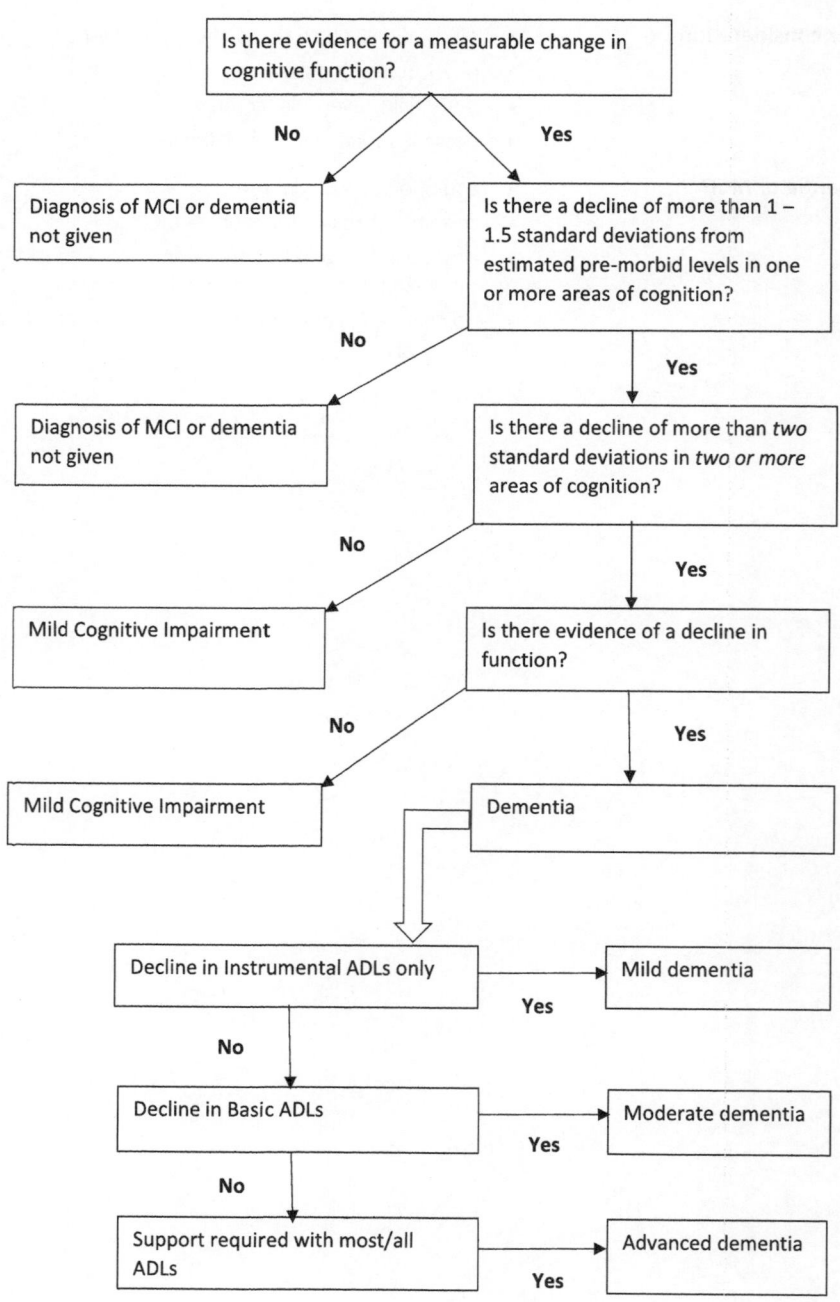

References

Albert, M. S., DeKosky, S. T., Dickson, D., et al. (2011). The diagnosis of mild cognitive impairment due to Alzheimer's disease: Recommendations from the National Institute on Aging-Alzheimer's Association workgroups on diagnostic guidelines for Alzheimer's disease. *Alzheimer's & Dementia: The Journal of the Alzheimer's Association*, 7(3), 270–9.

American Psychiatric Association (2013). *Diagnostic and Statistical Manual of Mental Disorders*, Fifth Edition, Text Revision. Washington, DC, American Psychiatric Association.

Antonelli Incalzi, R., Marra, C., Giordano, A., et al. (2003). Cognitive impairment in chronic obstructive pulmonary disease. *Journal of Neurology*, 250(3), 325–32.

Barnett, J. H., Blackwell, A. D., Sahakian, B. J., & Robbins, T. W. (2015). The Paired Associates Learning (PAL) test: 30 years of CANTAB translational neuroscience from laboratory to bedside in dementia research. In T. W. Robbins & B. J. Sahakian (Eds.), *Translational Neuropsychopharmacology: Current Topics in Behavioral Neurosciences* (pp. 449–74). Cham: Springer.

Bayer, A. J. (2018). The role of biomarkers and imaging in the clinical diagnosis of dementia. *Age and Ageing*, 47, 641–3.

Beach, T. G., Monsell, S. E., Phillips, L. E., & Kukull, W. (2012). Accuracy of the clinical diagnosis of Alzheimer disease at National Institute on Aging Alzheimer Disease Centers, 2005–2010. *Journal of Neuropathology & Experimental Neurology*, 71, 266–73.

Beynon, R., Sterne, J. A., Wilcock, G., et al. (2012). Is MRI better than CT for detecting a vascular component to dementia? A systematic review and meta-analysis. *BMC Neurology*, 12, 1–10.

Borson, S., Scanlan, J., Brush, M., Vitaliano, P., & Dokmak, A. (2000). The Mini-Cog: A cognitive 'vital signs' measure for dementia screening in multi-lingual elderly. *International Journal of Geriatric Psychiatry*, 15, 1021–7.

Boustani, M., Campbell, N., Munger, S., Maidment, I., & Fox, C. (2008). Impact of anticholinergics on the aging brain: A review and practical application. *Aging Health*, 4(3), 311–20.

Brodaty, H., Pond, D., Kemp, N. M., et al. (2002). The GPCOG: A new screening test for dementia designed for general practice. *Journal of the American Geriatrics Society*, 50 (3), 530–4.

Bucks, R., Ashworth, D., Wilcock, G., & Siegfried, K. (1996). Assessment of activities of daily living in dementia: development of the Bristol Activities of Daily Living Scale. *Age and Ageing*, 25, 113–20.

Clark, C. M., & Ewbank, D. C. (1996). Performance of the dementia severity rating scale: a caregiver questionnaire for rating severity in Alzheimer disease. *Alzheimer Disease and Associated Disorders*, 10(1), 31–9.

DeBettignies, B. H., Mahurin, R. K., & Pirozzolo, F. J. (1990). Insight for impairment in independent living skills in Alzheimer's disease and multi-infarct dementia. *Journal of Clinical and Experimental Neuropsychology*, 12, 355–63.

Elvevag, B., & Goldberg, T. E. (2000). Cognitive impairment in schizophrenia is the core of the disorder. *Critical Reviews in Neurobiology*, 14, 1–21.

Farias, S. T., Munga, S. D., Reed, B. R., et al. (2008). The measurement of everyday cognition (ECog): Scale development and psychometric properties. *Neuropsychology*, 22(4), 531–44.

Fisher, A. G. (1994). *Assessment of Motor and Processing Skill. Unpublished test manual.* Department of Occupational Therapy, Colorado State University, Fort Collins. CO.

Folstein, M. F., Folstein, S. E., & McHugh, P. R. (1975). Mini-mental state. A practical method for grading the cognitive state of patients for the clinician. *Journal of Psychiatric Research*, 12(3), 189–98.

Giebel, C. M., & Challis, D. (2017). Sensitivity of the mini-mental state examination, Montreal cognitive assessment and the Addenbrooke's cognitive examination III to everyday activity impairments in dementia: An exploratory study. *International Journal of Geriatric Psychiatry*, 32(10), 1085–93.

Harper, L., Barkhof, F., Scheltens, P., Schott, J., & Fox, N. (2014). An algorithmic approach to structural imaging in dementia. *Journal of Neurology, Neurosurgery and Psychiatry*, **85**, 692–8.

Hart, R. P., Wade, J. B., & Martelli, M. F. (2003). Cognitive impairment in patients with chronic pain: The significance of stress. *Current Science Inc*, **7**, 116–26.

Harvey, P. D., & Keefe, R. S. (2001). Studies of cognitive change in patients with schizophrenia following novel antipsychotic treatment. *American Journal of Psychiatry*, **158**(2), 176–84.

Hobus, P. P. M., Boshuizen, H. P. A., & Schmidt, H. G. (1990). Expert-novice differences in the role of contextual factors in early medical diagnosis. *Paper presented at the Annual Meeting of the American Educational Research Association* (Boston, MA, 16–20 April 1990).

Hodges, J. R., & Larner, A. J. (2017). Addenbrooke's Cognitive Examinations: ACE, ACE-R, ACE-III, ACEapp, and M-ACE. In A. J. Larner (Ed.) *Cognitive Screening Instruments: A Practical Approach, Second Edition*. Berlin: Springer, pp. 109–37.

Hsieh, S., Schubert, S., Hoon, C., Mioshi, E., & Hodges, J. R. (2013). Validation of the Addenbrooke's cognitive examination III in frontotemporal dementia and Alzheimer's disease. *Dementia and Geriatric Cognitive Disorders*, **36**(3–4), 242–50.

Jorm, A. F. (1994). A short from of the Informant Questionnaire on Cognitive Decline in the Elderly (QICODE): Development and cross-validation. *Psychological Medicine*, **24**(1), 145–53.

Jorm, A. F., Scott, R., & Jacomb, P. A. (1989). Assessment of cognitive decline in dementia by informant questionnaire. *International Journal of Geriatric Psychiatry*, **4**, 35–9.

Kalish, V. B., Gillham, J. E., & Unwin, B. K. (2014). Delirium in older persons: Evaluation and management. *American Family Physician*, **90**(3), 150–8.

Katzman, R., Brown, T., & Fuld, P., et al. (1983) Validation of a short orientation–memory–concentration test of cognitive impairment. *American Journal of Psychiatry*, **40**(6), 734–9.

Kolodner, J. (1983). Towards an understanding of the role of experience in the evolution form novice to expert. *International Journal of Man-Machine Studies*, **19**(5), 497–518.

Lenehan, M. E., Klekociuk, S. Z., & Summers, M. J. (2012). Absence of a relationship between subjective memory complaint and objective memory impairment in mild cognitive impairment (MCI): Is it time to abandon subjective memory complaint as an MCI diagnostic criterion? *International Psychogeriatrics*, **24**(9), 1505–14.

Lin, F. R., Metter, E. J., O'Brien, R. J., et al. (2011). Hearing loss and incident dementia. *Archives of Neurology*, **68**(2), 214–20.

Liu, C. M., & Lee, C. T. C. (2019). Association of hearing loss with dementia. *JAMA Network Open*, **2**(7), e198112.

Lodeiro-Fernández, L., Lorenzo-López, L., Maseda, A., et al. (2015). The impact of hearing loss on language performance in older adults with different stages of cognitive function. *Clinical Interventions in Aging*, 695–702.

MacKenzie, N. E., Kowalchuk, C., Agarwal, S. M., et al. (2018). Antipsychotics, metabolic adverse effects, *and cognitive function in schizophrenia. Frontiers in Psychiatry*, **9**, 622.

Macnamara, A., Schinazi, V. R., Chen, C., Coussens, S., & Loetscher, T. (2021). Vision impairments reduce cognitive test performance. *Nature Aging*, **1**, 975–6.

Mara, C., Cappa, A., & Fuso, L. (2003). Cognitive impairment in chronic obstructive pulmonary disease: A neuropsychological and spect study. *Journal of Neurology*, **250**(3), 325–32.

Mathuranath, P. S., Nestor, P. J., Berrio, G. E., Rakowicz, W., & Hodges, J. R. (2000). A brief cognitive test battery to differentiate Alzheimer's disease and frontotemporal dementia. *Neurology*, **55**(11), 1613–20.

McKeith, I. G., Boeve, B. F., & Dickson, D. W., et al. (2017). Diagnosis and management of dementia with Lewy bodies: Fourth consensus report of the DLB Consortium. *Neurology*, **89**, 88–100.

Merriam-Webster (2020). *Merriam-Webster's Dictionary and Thesaurus: Revised and Updated.* Springfield: *Merriam-Webster Incorporated.*

Moelter, S. T., Glenn, M. A., Xie, S. X., et al. (2015). The Dementia Severity Rating Scale predicts clinical dementia rating sum of boxes scores. *Alzheimer Disease and Associated Disorders, 29*(2), 158–60.

Nasreddine, Z. S., Phillips, N. A., Bédirian, V., et al. (2005). The Montreal Cognitive Assessment, MoCA: A brief screening tool for mild cognitive impairment. *Journal of the American Geriatrics Society, 53*(4), 695–9.

National Institute of Clinical Excellence (NICE) (2018). Dementia: Assessment, management and support for people living with dementia and their carers. https://www.nice.org.uk/guidance/ng97.

Orleans-Foley, S., Isaacs, J., & Cook, L. (2018). Neuroimaging for dementia diagnosis Guidance from the London Dementia Clinical Network. www.england.nhs.uk/london/wp-content/uploads/sites/8/2019/09/Neuroimaging-for-dementia-diagnosis-London-Dementia-Clinical-Network.pdf.

Parfenov, V. A., Zakharov, V. V., Kabaeva, A. R., & Vakhnina, N. V. (2020). Subjective cognitive decline as a predictor of future cognitive decline: A systematic review. *Dementia & Neuropsychologia, 14*(3), 248–57.

Pfeffer, R. I., Kurosaki, T. T., Harrah, C. H., Jr., et al. (1982). Measurement of functional activities in older adults in the community. *Journal of Gerontology, 37*(3), 323–9.

Rikkert, M. G., Tona, K. D., Janssen, L., et al. (2011). Validity, reliability, and feasibility of clinical staging scales in dementia: a systematic review. *American Journal of Alzheimer's Disease and Other Dementias, 26*(5), 357–65.

Salluh, J. I., Wang, H., Schneider, E. B., et al. (2015). Outcome of delirium in critically ill patients: systematic review and meta-analysis. *British Medical Journal (Clinical research ed.), 350*, h2538.

Schubert, C., Denmark, T. K., Crandall, B., Grome, A., & Pappas, J. (2013). Characterizing novice-expert differences in macrocognition: An exploratory study of cognitive work in the emergency department. *Annals of Emergency Medicine, 61*(1), 96–109.

Scott, J., Spector, A., Orrell, M., et al. (2017). Limited validity of the Hospital Anxiety and Depression Scale (HADS) in dementia: Evidence from a confirmatory factor analysis. *International Journal of Geriatric Psychiatry, 32*(7), 805–13.

Shin, S. Y., Katz, P., Wallhagen, M., & Julian, L. (2012). Cognitive impairment in persons with rheumatoid arthritis. *Arthritis Care & Research, 64*(8), 1144–50.

Siciliano, M., Chiorri, C., Passaniti, C., et al. (2019). Comparison of alternate and original forms of the Montreal Cognitive Assessment (MoCA): An Italian normative study. *Neurological Sciences, 40*(4), 691–702.

Tomaszewski Farias, S., Mungas, D., Harvey, D. J., et al. (2011). The measurement of everyday cognition: Development and validation of a short form of the Everyday Cognition scales. *Alzheimer's & Dementia, 7* (6), 593–601.

Vogels, R. L., Oosterman, J. M., Van Harten, B., et al. (2007). Profile of cognitive impairment in chronic heart failure. *Journal of the American Geriatrics Society, 55*(11), 1764–70.

Winblad, B., Palmer, K., Kivipelto, M., et al. (2004). Mild cognitive impairment – beyond controversies, towards a consensus: Report of the International Working Group on Mild Cognitive Impairment. *Journal of Internal Medicine, 256*(3), 240–6.

Zigmond, A. S., & Snaith, R. P. (1983). The hospital anxiety and depression scale. *Acta Psychiatrica Scandanavia, 67*, 361–70.

Chapter

3

Functional Neuroanatomy

Circuits: A General Principle of Brain Organisation

This chapter considers how the brain is organised, predominantly in terms of cognitive processing, with the aim of explaining terms used to describe cognition and relate this to how the systems break down in dementia. After various debates throughout the nineteenth and twentieth centuries regarding whether cognitive functions are localised to specific brain regions or are distributed, the current school of thought is that it represents a bit of both, with organisation in terms of circuits which encompass multiple anatomic regions. The process of mapping out circuits in the brain is known as connectomics and makes extensive use of functional and structural neural imaging. Fornito, Zalesky, and Breakspear (2015) outlined three mechanisms whereby damage in a particular area leads to dysfunction in other areas of the circuit: (1) Diaschisis (von Monakow, 1914) is a concept which has been applied widely in the study of stroke and refers to how damage to a specific area results in a loss of function in an anatomically remote area by disrupting a circuit. The effects of diaschisis are immediately apparent. (2) Transneuronal degeneration involves structural changes which occur over time and affects areas remote from the original area. (3) Dedifferentiation refers to the recruitment of diffuse non-specific brain regions in the performance of cognitive tasks, which can result in circuits with reduced efficiency.

Neurons, Axons, and Dendrites

Neurons are the cells which form the communication networks in the human body. The brain is the 'control centre' where most of the neurons are concentrated, but their connections spread via the spinal cord and throughout the body. The soma is the cell body, and the axon is the connection which sends electrical impulses (action potentials) to other neurons. Dendrites are the connections whereby input is received from other neurons. When a charge reaches the end of an axon, it triggers the release of a chemical (neurotransmitter) via a junction with the dendrites of the next cell: this is called a synapse. Collectively, the signals coming into the neuron alter its charge, and when it reaches a particular threshold it fires an action potential. The circuits operate via this constant combination of electrical and chemical messages. An illustration of a neuron is seen in Figure 3.1.

In addition to neurons, the nervous system has a diverse range of glial cells, serving different functions. Although they play a role in transmission and communication, they do not generate electricity. Axons are insulated by a coating of myelin, which is a form of glial cell. The myelin has frequent gaps, known as Nodes of Ranvier, and the electrical charge jumps from gap to gap, which is known as saltatory conduction. If there is damage to the myelin, the axon will not be insulated properly and will no longer conduct the charge, which

34

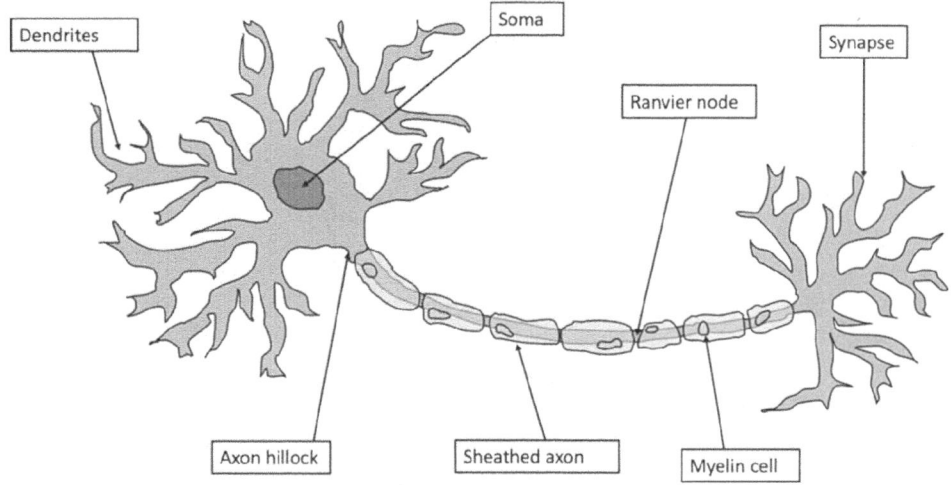

Figure 3.1 Example of a neuron. Example of a neuron © BrunelloN (https://commons.wikimedia.org/wiki/File:Ex ample_of_a_neuron.png). CC BY-SA 4.0 DEED.

can cause cognitive and motor problems according to where the demyelination has occurred. The most well-known example of a disease where this happens is multiple sclerosis, where the person's immune system attacks the myelin. In the relapsing-remitting form, as the immune system response subsides remyelination can occur, accompanied by a recovery of function. Slightly less well-known as a disorder which involves demyelination, alcohol-related brain damage (ARBD) is thought to involve two mechanisms which contribute to cognitive decline. Wernicke–Korsakoff's syndrome is related to vitamin B deficiency, and can cause irreversible damage. However, in addition to this, ethanol-related neurotoxicity is thought to exert an effect by causing demyelination, and the considerable improvement in cognitive ability which is often observed with sustained abstention from alcohol use may arise from remyelination (Arts, Wallvoort, & Kessels, 2017).

Grey Matter and White Matter

The terms 'grey matter' and 'white matter' refer to cell bodies and axons, which appear differently on scans. Cell bodies are concentrated in the cortex, which is the layer around the outside of the brain, and in the centre of the brain in a set of nuclei known collectively as the basal ganglia and thalamus. Figure 3.2 shows the position of these in relation to the cortex. The basal ganglia has traditionally been thought of as three structures: the caudate nucleus, the globus pallidus, and the putamen. More recent models have also included the substantia nigra, nucleus accumbens, and subthalamic nuclei (Simonyan, 2019). The amygdala, which sits at the end of the tail of the caudate nucleus, is anatomically part of the basal ganglia, but is considered separate as it has a different function. The thalamus acts as a relay station, through which multiple cognitive functions operate. Consequently, a strategic lesion to the thalamus can result in a diffuse pattern of impairment affecting multiple aspects of cognition.

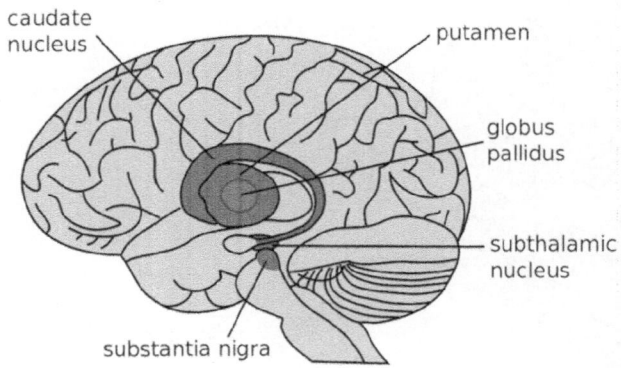

Figure 3.2 Basal ganglia in relation to the cortex. Basal Ganglia lateral © Badseed (https://commons.wikimedia.org/wiki/File:Basal_Ganglia_lateral.svg). Public domain.

The proposed role of the basal ganglia has evolved considerably, from being one of simply mediating aspects of motor control (Albin, Young, & Penney, 1989) to include roles in cognition, emotion (Florio et al., 2018), and psychiatric disorders (Macpherson & Hikida, 2019). The links between the basal ganglia and areas of the cortex, the thalamus, and the cerebellum has led to the use of the term 'circuit disorders' to describe movement disorders such as Parkinson's disease and psychiatric disorders such as Tourettes, obsessive-compulsive disorder, and depression (DeLong & Wichmann, 2010).

The Cortex

The way the cortex has been viewed over the last two centuries has changed along with most other views of brain function. It consists of the outermost layer of the brain and is a concentration of cell bodies in six layers. Although it was initially thought to simply be the 'covering' of the brain and not particularly important, it was subsequently mapped out extensively in terms of the function of specific regions (e.g. Brodman, 1909; Penfield & Boldrey, 1937). These maps have tended to allocate functions to discrete cortical areas, and are still used (Strotzer, 2009). Things have continued to evolve since then to view function in terms of circuits, and also to take account of the role of subcortical areas such as the basal ganglia, thalamus, and cerebellum. Figure 3.3 shows a typical map of the cortex, with motor and sensory functions assigned.

There are some general principals of cerebral organisation. In very simple terms, the back of the brain is concerned with input, and the front of the brain is concerned with output. The primary visual cortex is located in the occipital lobe, auditory information is processed via the temporal lobe, and sensory information is integrated via the parietal lobe. The motor cortex is located in the frontal lobe, which is directly anterior to the primary sensory cortex in the parietal lobe. The prefrontal cortex is concerned with executive function, encompassing skills such as planning, reasoning, and decision-making. Although it is usually said that memory is based in the temporal lobe, this is best considered in terms of a circuit involving multiple areas, in the same way as executive function is considered in terms of circuits between the prefrontal cortex and basal ganglia.

Another general principal of organisation is lateralisation. The cortex is divided into two hemispheres, with most aspects of language function based in the left and visual-spatial

Motor and Sensory Regions of the Cerebral Cortex

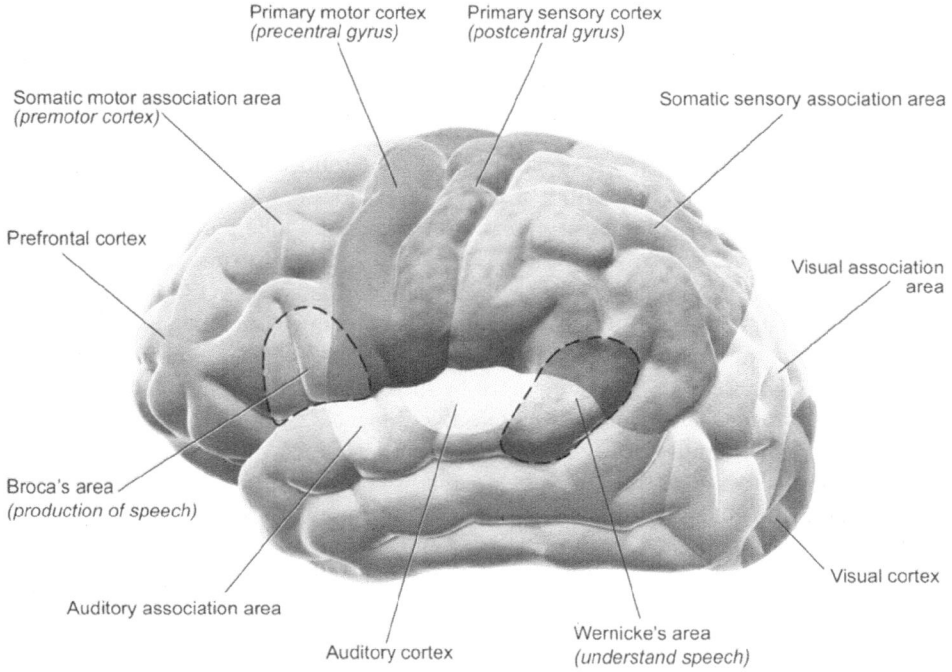

Figure 3.3 Motor and sensory regions of the cortex. Blausen.com staff (2014). "Medical gallery of Blausen Medical 2014". WikiJournal of Medicine 1(2). DOI:10.15347/wjm/2014.010. ISSN 2002-4436

function concentrated in the right. However, the degree of lateralisation can vary considerably between people, and some people show the reverse pattern of lateralisation with language function concentrated in the right hemisphere.

Cognitive Processes and Associated Circuits

Although there are ongoing debates about the precise meaning of the word 'cognition', often from a philosophical perspective or in relation to whether non-human species demonstrate true cognitive abilities (e.g. Bayne et al., 2019), it is necessary to be pragmatic and work with an operational definition. For this book, the definition of cognition will be the original one put forward by Neisser (1967, p. 4) of 'all processes by which sensory input is transformed, reduced, elaborated, stored, recovered and used'. This typically includes the following processes: attention, memory, perception, language, and executive function. Whilst I argue in Chapter 1 that it is also important to measure speed of information processing, this is not a specific form of cognition, but a general property which is often highly sensitive to brain dysfunction. Although there was a tradition of considering emotion/affect as separate to cognition, this distinction is less frequently maintained now, and it can be argued that emotion/affect meets Neisser's definition of cognition (Duncan & Barret, 2007). It makes sense to start with the most basic cognitive processes and work up to the most complex.

Perception

Sensation/sensory information refers to the output of our sensory organs, and is traditionally classified as vision, hearing, smell, taste, and touch. In addition to these, the brain receives information about body position, movement, balance, pain, and temperature. Perception is how the brain processes this information.

Visual perception has been extensively researched, with scrutiny of other modalities developing more recently. Basic visual information is processed within the visual cortex in the occipital lobes, after which it is processed by two anatomically distinct circuits referred to as the dorsal stream and the ventral stream (Ungerleider & Mishkin, 1982). The dorsal stream forms a circuit via the sensory areas and the parietal lobes, and is responsible for spatial processing (i.e. where things are). The ventral stream forms a circuit from the sensory areas via the temporal lobes and is responsible for object recognition and allocating meaning. Although initially proposed as circuits for processing visual information, it is now considered that other cognitive processes such audition, language comprehension and production, and attention are also supported by these circuits (Cloutman, 2013).

The dorsal and ventral streams can be selectively affected by brain injury and degenerative disorders. An example of a degenerative disorder which initially affects the dorsal stream without affecting the ventral stream is posterior cortical atrophy (PCA) (McMonagle et al., 2006). This is usually an atypical presentation of Alzheimer's disease, which leads to atrophy in the occipito-parietal region and early visuospatial difficulties such as being unable to locate, reach for, and interpret objects under visual guidance (Crutch et al., 2017). There are often difficulties with judging distance, which can sometimes lead to accidents whilst driving, such as mounting the kerb, and problems with parking.

The opposite pattern of selective impairment to the ventral stream can be seen in semantic variant primary progressive aphasia (svPPA), which is characterised by anteroinferior and mesial temporal lobe atrophy and can present with an inability to recognise objects by sight if the atrophy is concentrated in the left hemisphere (agnosia) or familiar faces if concentrated in the right hemishphere (prosopagnosia) (Marshall et al., 2018).

Language

The identification of different forms of language disorder associated with damage to different brain areas represented the earliest evidence of localisation of function. In most people, most language functions are based in the left hemisphere, although some people can show a reversal of this pattern (Basso et al., 1985), and in some people the degree of lateralisation is not so strong (Chance & Crow, 2007). Even in typically lateralised people, some aspects of language comprehension are carried out by the right hemisphere, such as prosody (interpreting meaning from patterns of stress and intonation), pictographic reading (information represented through pictures), and appreciation of metaphors (Taylor & Regard, 2003).

Comprehension and production of single words and sentences, and the rules for how words are combined in a meaningful way (syntax), are carried out by the left hemisphere in most people. Expressive language is associated with an anterior system, located towards the posterior end of the left frontal lobes, and comprehension is associated with the left posterior-parietal area (Scott & Schoenberg, 2012). Damage to the anterior system can result in an expressive dysphasia (Broca's aphasia) characterised by difficulty with speech production, speech creation, and comprehension of syntax. Damage to the posterior system is associated with fluent, but often meaningless, speech production and impaired speech comprehension (Wernicke's aphasia). See Figure 3.3 for a diagram of where these areas are located. A disconnection between these systems can result in a pattern of some speech production errors, reasonably preserved comprehension, but seriously impaired speech repetition (Swanberg et al., 2007).

Memory

Before looking at the circuits involved in episodic memory, it is worth clarifying some of the terminology relating to the cognitive processes involved. Episodic memory refers to recall of events, which means things with some form of time reference. Virtually all forms of memory test (e.g. list learning, story recall, visual reproduction) assess episodic memory because they are testing for recall of something the person was exposed to at a particular time. Semantic memory is the permanent repository for facts you have learned, where information can ultimately be stored. In a fully functioning brain, episodic memory and semantic memory both operate and interact, but following lesions to the relevant circuits, you can find that one system is greatly impaired whilst the other still functions.

Another very important distinction is between the processes of encoding, storage, and retrieval. Encoding is the process of creating a memory, and is the equivalent of pressing a 'record' button. Retrieval refers to the ability to access the stored information when required (play). Storage is the ability to keep the information once it has been encoded. It is possible to have deficits in all of these processes, but typically an organic memory disorder is most likely to affect encoding (i.e. creating new memories). Inability to create new memories following an illness or injury is referred to as anterograde amnesia. Retrograde amnesia refers to an inability to recall items/events from the period before and leading up to the onset of illness/injury.

The classic memory circuit, which was originally thought to carry out emotional processing, was the Papez circuit (Papez, 1937). There have been various additions to this circuit, and it was also renamed the limbic system and incorporated into the concept of the triune brain (Maclean, 1990). The Papez circuit is outlined in Figure 3.4. The significance of this circuit for episodic memory came to be realised following a number of cases studies of people developing anterograde amnesia following damage to structures in this circuit, for example the fornix (Wang et al., 2018), the hippocampus (Milner & Scoville, 1957), mamillary bodies (Dusoir et al., 1990). The hub of this circuit has been traced to a specific part of the hippocampus called the subiculum, where it joins with the retrosplenial cortex. In a study of 53 amnesiacs, only two did not have involvement of this area (Ferguson et al., 2019).

The Papez circuit is concerned with the basic activity of creating new memories, and is based in the medial temporal lobes. Semantic memory, which is a permanent repository, is a distributed, multi-modal process, co-ordinated and integrated via a convergence zone (Damasio, 1989). The temporal pole, which is the most anterior part of the temporal lobe (see Figure 3.5) has been considered the most likely location for the semantic memory convergence zone as it is the area most frequently implicated in the development of semantic dementia (Gorno-Tempini et al., 2011), although the exact location and whether this is something carried out bilaterally or based primarily in the left hemisphere has been questioned (Tsapkini, Frangakis, & Hillis, 2011). Linked in with this extended circuit, the

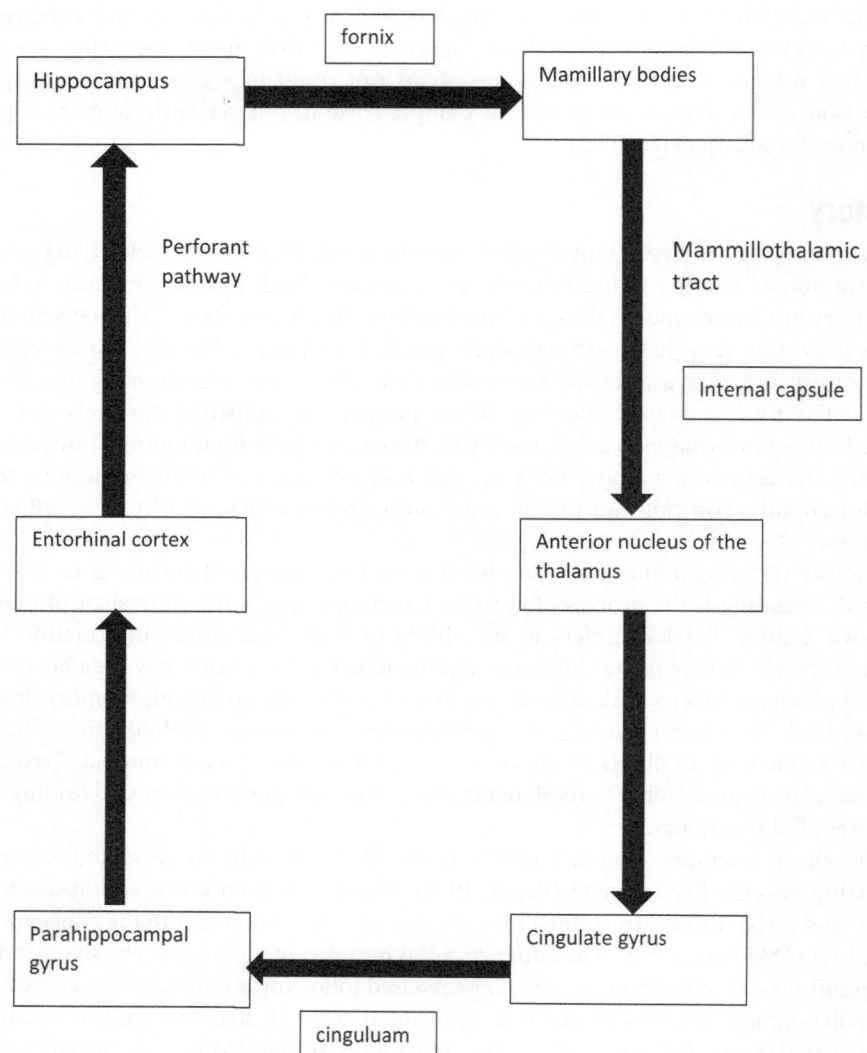

Figure 3.4 Original structures thought to be involved in the Papez circuit

role of the frontal lobes in memory has developed considerably in recent decades. Whilst acknowledging that the range of mechanism is constantly being refined, there is some agreement that the frontal systems contribute to the organisation of memory and encoding and retrieval of information in episodic memory (Lee, Robbins, & Owen, 2000).

Attention

The American Psychological Association Dictionary of Psychology defines attention as 'a state in which cognitive resources are focused on certain aspects of the environment rather than on others and the central nervous system is in a state of readiness to respond to stimuli' (https://dictionary.apa.org/attention). One of the most influential models of human

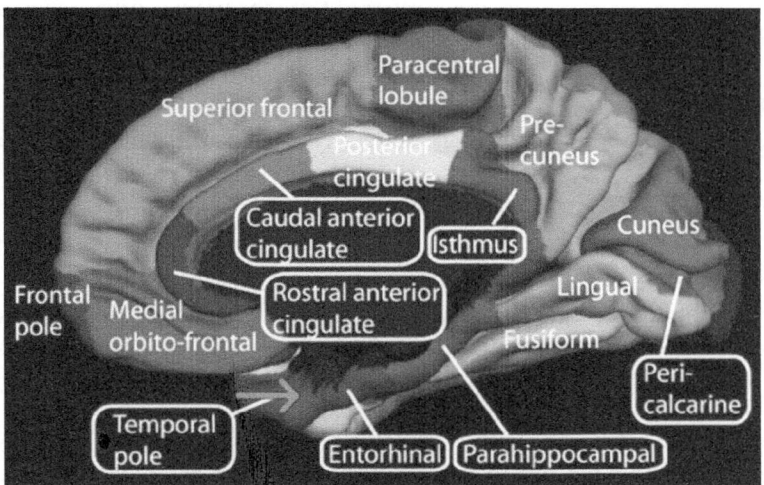

Figure 3.5 Sagittal view of the brain, illustrating the locations of the dorsolateral prefrontal cortex, orbitofrontal cortex and cingulate cortex. Hagmann P, Cammoun L, Gigandet X, Meuli R, Honey CJ, et al. (2008). Mapping the Structural Core of Human Cerebral Cortex. *PLoS Biol* 6(7): e159. doi:10.1371/journal.pbio.0060159. CC BY 2.5 DEED.

attention was put forward by Posner and Petersen (1990), updated in Petersen and Posner (2012). Attention is divided into three networks:

1) Alerting. This consists of maintaining levels of arousal and alertness. Arousal is associated with the brain stem, and alertness is associated with the right hemisphere.
2) Orienting. This is the process of prioritising sensory input and is associated with the parietal cortex.
3) Executive. This is associated with midline frontal and anterior cingulate areas.

Models of attention overlap to some degree with models of executive function, although there are enough distinct elements to mean the two terms are not interchangeable.

Executive Function

'Executive function' is an umbrella term covering the highest levels of cognitive processing, which includes skills such as reasoning, problem solving, planning, and decision-making. Motor, cognitive, and emotional functions are supported by circuits between the frontal lobes and basal ganglia (fronto-striatal circuits), which also connect to the thalamus (Alexander & Crutcher, 1999). The original model described five fronto-striatal circuits: motor, oculomotor, dorsolateral, orbital, and anterior cingulate. The non-motor circuits are thought to support the following functions:

1. Dorsolateral prefrontal circuit is involved in the aspects of cognitive processing measured by neuropsychological testing (e.g. set-shifting, generativity, response inhibition, problem solving, working memory).
2. Orbitofrontal circuit is involved in social cognition, judgement, and mood. Damage to this pathway can give rise to behavioural disinhibition, socially inappropriate behaviour, and poor decision-making.

3. Anterior cingulate cortex, sometimes referred to as the limbic cortex, is involved in initiation of behaviour. Damage to this circuit can lead to apathy.

The cingulate gyrus has been associated with the concept of self-regulation/self-control, with the dorsal cingulate gyrus being related to cognitive tasks (Botvinick et al., 2001) and the ventral cingulate gyrus being more closed associated with emotion (Bush, Luu, & Posner, 2000).

The locations of these areas are illustrated in Figure 3.5.

Emotion/Affect

The study of emotions was curiously absent from much of the development of psychology as a science. This has to some extent been redressed over the last three decades, with an increased understanding of what is meant by emotions and how these are processed via a number of distributed networks.

Emotion and cognition are intertwined in the brain. The amygdala, for example, is involved in processing emotional stimuli, and its interactions with prefrontal regions influence decision-making and memory. The ventromedial prefrontal cortex is important for integrating emotional and cognitive information during decision-making.

Cognition and emotion interact, with structures such as the amygdala being involved in processing of emotional stimuli, and creating associations which underlie anxiety (LeDoux, 1996). The ventromedial prefrontal cortex integrates emotion and executive processing to contribute towards efficient decision-making (Damasio, 1999).

A comprehensive review of the neuropsychology of emotion is beyond the scope of this book, and possibly of limited clinical relevance as models of emotion have yet to be extensively incorporated into clinical diagnosis of dementia.

Key Points

- There have been many debates regarding whether the brain is organised according to localised or distributed function. The current school of thought incorporates elements of both by considering the brain in terms of areas of localised function contributing to circuits distributed across different anatomical regions.
- The most basic units of communication are called neurons, which consist of cell bodies and interconnections.
- The cell bodies are referred to as grey matter, and the connections are white matter, based upon their different appearance on scans.
- Grey matter is concentrated in the cortex and subcortical areas known as the basal ganglia. These are connected by white matter.
- Perceptual processes deal with the input from sensory organs. Vision is concentrated towards the back of the brain, in the occipital lobe.
- Hearing is processed in the temporal lobes, where most aspects of memory are also based.
- The frontal lobes deal with output, including control of movement and executive functions such as planning and decision-making.
- Emotion and cognition are interlinked, and processing in one domain is influenced by the other.

References

Albin, R. L., Young, A. B., & Penney, J. B. (1989). The functional anatomy of basal ganglia disorders. *Trends in Neurosciences*, **12**(10), 366–75.

Alexander, G. E., & Crutcher, M. D. (1990). Functional architecture of basal ganglia circuits: Neural substrates of parallel processing. *Trends in Neurosciences*, **13**(7), 266–271.

Arts, N., Walvoort, S., & Kessels, R. (2017). Korsakoff's syndrome: A critical review. *Neuropsychiatric Disease and Treatment*, **13**, 2875–90.

Basso, A., Capitani, E., Laiacona, M., & Zanobio, M. E. (1985). Crossed aphasia: One or more syndromes? *Cortex*, **21**(1), 25–45.

Bayne, T., Brainard, D., Byrne, R. W., et al. (2019). What is cognition? *Current Biology*, **29**(13), R608–R615.

Botvinick, M. M., Braver, T. S., Barch, D. M., Carter, C. S., & Cohen, J. D. (2001). Conflict monitoring and cognitive control. *Psychological Review*, **108**(3), 624.

Brodmann, K. (1909). *Vergleichende Lokalisationslehre der Großhirnrinde in ihren Prinzipien dargestellt auf Grund des Zellenbaues*. Leipzig: Barth.

Bush, G., Luu, P., & Posner, M. I. (2000). Cognitive and emotional influences in anterior cingulate cortex. *Trends in Cognitive Sciences*, **4**(6), 215–22.

Chance, S. A., & Crow, T. J. (2007). Distinctively human: Cerebral lateralisation and language in Homo sapiens. *Journal of Anthropological Science*, **85**, 83–100.

Cloutman, L. L. (2013). Interaction between dorsal and ventral processing streams: where, when and how?. *Brain and Language*, **127**(2), 251–63.

Crutch, S. J., Schott, J. M., Rabinovici, G. D., et al. (2017). Consensus classification of posterior cortical atrophy. *Alzheimer's & Dementia*, **13**(8), 870–84.

Damasio, A. R. (1989). The brain binds entities and events by multiregional activation from convergence zones. *Neural Computation*, **1**(1), 123–32.

Damasio, A. R. (1999). *The Feeling of What Happens: Body and Emotion in the Making of Consciousness*. New York: Harcourt.

DeLong, M., & Wichmann, T. (2010). Changing views of basal ganglia circuits and circuit disorders. *Clinical EEG and Neuroscience*, **41**(2), 61–7.

Duncan, S., & Barrett, L. F. (2007). Affect is a form of cognition: A neurobiological analysis. *Cognition and Emotion*, **21**(6), 1184–211.

Dusoir, H., Kapur, N., Byrnes, D. P., McKinstry, S., & Hoare, R. D. (1990). The role of diencephalic pathology in human memory disorder: Evidence from a penetrating paranasal brain injury. *Brain*, **113**(6), 1695–706.

Ferguson, M. A., Lim, C., Cooke, D., et al. (2019). A human memory circuit derived from brain lesions causing amnesia. *Nature Communications*, **10**(1), 1–9.

Florio, T. M., Scarnati, E., Rosa, I., et al. (2018). The basal ganglia: More than just a switching device. *CNS Neuroscience & therapeutics*, **24**(8), 677–84.

Fornito, A., Zalesky, A., & Breakspeare, M. (2015). The connectomics of brain disorders. *Nature Reviews: Neuroscience*, **16**, 159–72.

Gorno-Tempini, M. L., Hillis, A. E., Weintraub, S., et al. (2011). Classification of primary progressive aphasia and its variants. *Neurology*, **76**(11), 1006–14.

LeDoux, J. (1996). *The Emotional Brain*. New York; Simon & Schuster.

Lee, A., Robbins, T. W., & Owen, A. M. (2000). Episodic memory meets working memory in the frontal lobe: Functional neuroimaging studies of encoding and retrieval. *Critical Reviews in Neurobiology*, **14**(3–4), 165–97.

MacLean, P. D. (1990). *The Triune Brain in Evolution: Role in Paleocerebral Functions*. New York: Springer Science & Business Media.

Macpherson, T., & Hikida, T. (2019). Role of basal ganglia neurocircuitry in the pathology of psychiatric disorders. *Psychiatry and Clinical Neurosciences*, **73**(6), 289–301.

Marshall, C. R., Hardy, C. J., Volkmer, A., et al. (2018). Primary progressive aphasia: a clinical approach. *Journal of Neurology*, **265**(6), 1474–90.

McMonagle, P., Deering, F., Berliner, Y., & Kertesz, A. (2006). The cognitive profile of posterior cortical atrophy. *Neurology*, **66**(3), 331–8.

Milner, B., & Scoville, W. (1957). Loss of recent memory after bilateral hippocampal lesions. *The Journal of Neurology, Neurosurgery and Psychiatry*, **20**, 11–21.

Neisser, U. (1967). *Cognitive Psychology*. New York: Appleton-Century-Crofts.

Papez, J. W. (1937). A proposed mechanism of emotion. *Archives of Neurology and Psychiatry*, **38**, 725–43.

Penfield, W., & Boldrey, E. (1937). Somatic motor and sensory representation in the cerebral cortex of man as studied by electrical stimulation. *Brain*, **60**(4), 389–443.

Petersen, S. E., & Posner, M. I. (2012). The attention system of the human brain: 20 years after. *Annual Review of Neuroscience*, **35**, 73–89.

Posner, M. I., & Petersen, S. E. (1990). The attention system of the human brain. *Annual Review of Neuroscience*, **13**(1), 25–42.

Scott, J. G., & Schoenberg, M. R. (2012). Language problems and assessment: The aphasic patient. In M. R. Schoenberg & J. G. Scott (Eds.), *The Little Black Book of Neuropsychology* (pp. 159–78). New York: Springer.

Simonyan, K. (2019). Recent advances in understanding the role of the basal ganglia. *F1000Research*, **8**.

Strotzer, M. (2009). One century of brain mapping using Brodmann areas. *Clinical Neuroradiology*, **19**(3), 179–86.

Swannberg, M. M., Nasreddine, Z. S., Meendez, M. F., & Cummings, J. L. (2007). Speech and Language. In C. G. Goetz (Ed.), *Textbook of Clinical Neurology*, vol 35 (pp. 79–98). Philadelphia: Elsevier Health Sciences.

Taylor, K. I., & Regard, M. (2003). Language in the right cerebral hemisphere: Contributions from reading studies. *Physiology*, **18**(6), 257–61.

Tsapkini, K., Frangakis, C., & Hillis, A. E. (2011). The function of the left anterior temporal pole: Evidence from acute stroke and infarct volume. *Brain*, **134**(10), 3094–105.

Ungerleider, L. G., & Mishkin, M. (1982). Two cortical visual systems. In D. J. Ingle, M. A. Goodale, & R. J. W. Mansfield (Eds.), *Analysis of Visual Behavior* (pp. 549–86). Cambridge, MA: MIT Press.

von Monakow C. (1914). *Die Localization im Grosshirn und der Abbau der Funktion durch korticale Herde*. Wiesbaden: J. F. Bergmann.

Wang, J., Ke, J., Zhou, C., & Yin, C. (2018). Amnesia due to the injury of papez circuit following isolated fornix column infarction. *Journal of Stroke and Cerebrovascular Diseases*, **27**(5), 1431–3.

Neuropsychological Assessment in Dementia Diagnosis

This chapter aims to explain some of the concepts underlying neuropsychology in an accessible manner, based upon many years of teaching and training neuropsychologists, clinical psychologists, and other professionals. Consequently, this chapter is likely to be the most subjective chapter in this book.

Who Can Undertake a Neuropsychological Assessment?

It is important to remember that the different professions involved in multi-disciplinary team diagnosis have different areas of emphasis in their training, and neuropsychological assessment does not feature in the core training of any profession other than clinical psychologists. This is not to say that a member of another profession has not undertaken further training in neuropsychology, but it is not covered extensively in the basic training of medics (including psychiatrists, neurologists, and geriatricians), nurses, occupational therapists, speech and language therapists, or physiotherapists. It is also important to realise that whilst some clinical psychologists have a basic grounding in psychometric testing and may have extensive knowledge of applying that in their area of work, this is not equivalent to the considerably more extensive specialised training required to be a neuropsychologist. However, I would not wish to advocate that only a neuropsychologist can undertake a neuropsychological assessment for dementia. In fact, a practitioner psychologist with an appropriate grounding in neuropsychology and working within a dementia assessment service should be appropriately positioned to do so. The material chosen for this chapter bears this in mind and is not intended solely for qualified neuropsychologists.

When Is a Neuropsychological Assessment Required?

The most basic answer to this is when it is uncertain whether an individual has experienced a decline in cognitive function based on the data available so far. For many people, a score considerably below threshold on a cognitive screening instrument within the context of the overall clinical presentation is sufficient to determine that some cognitive decline has occurred. In fact, in such cases further cognitive testing is unlikely to be informative and possibly unethical as unnecessary investigations may result in patient distress. However, in other cases, such as those with unusual initial presentations, or people whose premorbid abilities were likely to have fallen some way above or below average, a neuropsychological assessment may be the best way to confirm or disconfirm whether there has been any change and possibly identify what underlies the presentation.

Assumptions Underlying Neuropsychological Assessment

There are a number of assumptions which underlie neuropsychological assessment, many of which are now considered to be only loosely correct. This is not intended as a criticism of the profession, as the same is also true of many other areas of medical assessment. It is, however, important to realise and acknowledge that the approach has certain limitations.

1. Localisation of function. This is the assumption that different cognitive functions are localised to specific areas of the brain, following on from which evidence of cognitive decline should be reflected in patterns of atrophy seen on scans. Whilst there is a degree of functional cognitive architecture from which conclusions may be drawn (e.g. input is concentrated in the back of the brain, output in the front, language function is predominantly located in the brain's left hemisphere, whereas visual-spatial functions are located in the right), this is not absolute. Some people show atypical patterns of lateralisation, and cognitive functions tend to operate in distributed networks spanning more than one brain region.

2) The theory of modularity (Fodor, 1983) was highly influential, particularly in the field of cognitive neuropsychology (Ellis & Young, 1988). This is the idea that the brain is organised into discrete, functionally separate processing units which can be selectively damaged, leaving others functionally intact. Although the approach has had its critics (e.g. Plaut, 1995), the assumption that some functions can be impaired whilst others remain intact has always been central to neuropsychology. In clinical practice, however, such clear distinctions are less common than patterns of relative strengths and weaknesses.

3) As some abilities remain intact following brain damage or illness, it is possible to use these abilities to estimate premorbid ability. It is also possible to use demographic variables, which are by definition premorbid. The discrepancy between current scores and estimated premorbid ability scores can be used to determine if there has been a decline in cognitive function. Whilst this is one of the great strengths of neuropsychology, and makes the approach more powerful than using a screening test with a fixed cut-off score, every method of estimating premorbid ability has its limitations and there will always be unusual cases where an accurate estimate of premorbid ability is highly challenging.

4) Ecological validity – the ability to predict everyday function. Whilst cognitive ability and everyday function should be related, cognitive tests can be notoriously poor predictors of everyday function.

Psychometrics

Psychometrics refers to the *quantitative* measurement of psychological processes and behaviour. Whilst qualitative information will always be a major part of any psychological assessment, quantitative measurement is at the core of neuropsychology. Psychometrics makes extensive use of statistics, and many statistical techniques have been developed within the context of measuring psychological processes. Whilst screening instruments often make use of a single cut-off score, neuropsychology incorporates a considerably more complex process of considering the probability of a particular score or scores occurring (i.e. how unusual it is). The important thing to appreciate is that any cognitive score on its own is meaningless – it only becomes useful when you compare it to other scores.

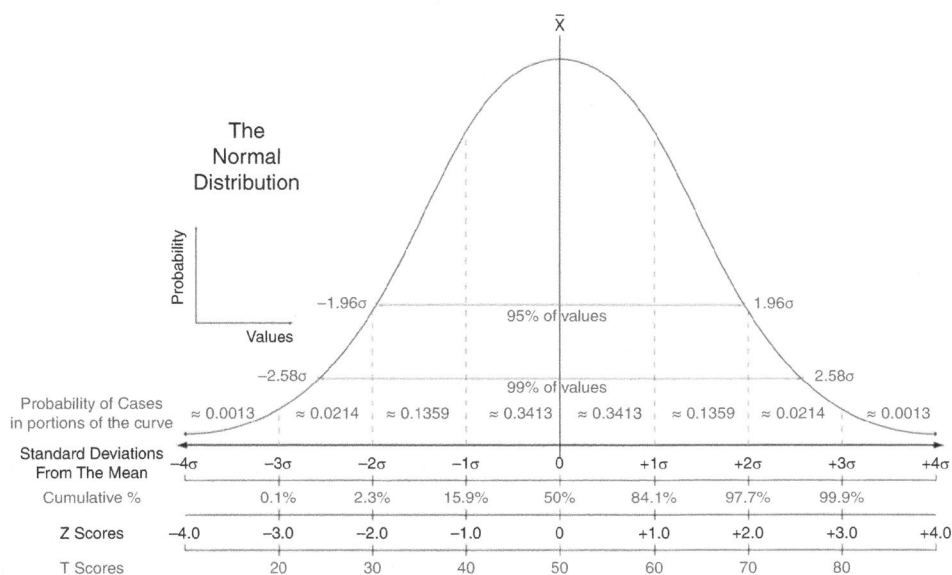

Figure 4.1 The normal distribution, showing the relationship between standard deviations, z scores, and T scores. The Normal Distribution © Heds 1 (https://commons.wikimedia.org/wiki/File:The_Normal_Distribution.svg). Public domain.

In order to understand this further, it is necessary to consider the 'normal' distribution, so called because it describes the way in which most naturally occurring characteristics you can measure are distributed. This includes things such as height, weight, lung capacity, foot size, and cognitive abilities. The key principle of the normal distribution is that most scores are clustered around the middle, with an increasingly small number of people showing very high or very low scores. An illustration of the normal distribution is shown in Figure 4.1.

To understand how this is applied requires some knowledge of a few basic statistical concepts. Although a neuropsychologist would be expected to have a more in-depth knowledge of statistics, I would argue that only a few concepts are required for a basic understanding of how statistics are used. More complex statistics are either a development from or a combination of these basic ideas.

1. **The average.** This refers to the central value of a set of numbers. There are different ways to calculate this, depending on the type of data being looked at. For psychometric assessment, the type of calculation used most will be the 'mean'. This is all the numbers in a group added together and then divided by how many were in the group. The mean is used when scores are interval data, which means that each point on a scale has an equal interval between them. If scores are put in order, irrespective of whether the difference between them is equal or not, this is called ordinal data. The average is calculated by putting all the scores in order and picking the one in the middle, which is called the 'median'. In a normal distribution of scores, the mean and median will be in the same place. To illustrate the difference between interval and ordinal data, a score of eight will always be twice the size of a score of four, as this is interval data. However, with ordinal data, where we deal with the position of scores when put in order, the score in eighth position is not necessarily twice the size of the score in fourth position.

2. **Standard deviation.** This is a measure of how spread out the scores are around the mean. A small standard deviation means the scores are clustered tightly around the mean, whereas a larger standard deviation means they are more spread out.
3. **Correlation.** This is a figure which tells you how closely two or more sets of measurements are related. For example, height and foot size are highly correlated as taller people have larger feet. A correlation coefficient of 1 means there is a perfect relationship, whereas 0 means there is no relationship.

Types of Scores

When a test is administered, this gives a set of raw scores, which tell us very little. To take on some meaning, they need to be compared to how everyone else has done on that test. When a test is designed it is standardised by giving it to a large number of people (the standardisation sample) and calculating the mean and standard deviation for all the scores. To give raw scores some meaning, they are converted into standard scores, of which there are several variants, all of which are calculated by comparing the score achieved to the mean and the standard deviation of the standardisation sample. The standardised score will tell you how many standard deviations the raw score was from the mean. The most basic example of a standardised score is a z score, covered in all basic statistical textbooks, which has a mean of 0 and a standard deviation of 1. So, a z score of +1 is one standard deviation above the mean, and a z score of −1 is one standard deviation below the mean. However, dealing with positive and negative numbers gets confusing, so in clinical practice a number of other types of standard score are used which are easier to understand. Whilst it is important to understand the logic behind different standard scores, we will not describe how to calculate them as clinical tests provide conversion tables in their manuals to allow you to look them up. Table 4.1 gives examples of different standard scores which may be encountered.

IQ tests, such as the Wechsler Adult Intelligence Scale (Wechsler, 2008), feature a number of different subtests, which are averaged together to give an overall IQ score. Index scores follow a similar logic, but are based on collections of subtests which are thought to measure similar underlying abilities, rather than averaging everything together. Index scores are more commonly used in neuropsychology than IQ scores as we are interested in identifying patterns of strengths and weaknesses rather than overall ability. Individual subtests are converted to scaled scores, which usually range from 1 to 19; however, there are exceptions, such as the Hayling and Brixton tests (Burgess & Shallice, 1997) which use scaled scores from 1 to 9. T scores use the same logic as index scores, but with a mean of 50 and a standard deviation of 10: these are less commonly found in test manuals.

Table 4.1 Standard scores which are likely to be encountered in clinical practice

Score	Type of data	Mean	Standard deviation
IQ score	Interval	100	15
Index score	Interval	100	15
Scaled score	Interval	10	3
T scores	Interval	50	10
Percentiles	Ordinal	50	n/a

Table 4.2 Corresponding index scores, scaled scores, percentiles, and classifications

IQ/Index score	Scaled score	Percentile	Wechsler Classification
145	19	99.9	Very Superior
140	18	99.6	Very Superior
135	17	99	Very Superior
130	16	98	Very Superior
125	15	95	Superior
120	14	91	Superior
115	13	84	High Average
110	12	75	High Average
105	11	63	Average
100	10	50	Average
95	9	37	Average
90	8	25	Average
85	7	16	Low Average
80	6	9	Low Average
75	5	5	Borderline
70	4	2	Borderline
65	3	1	Extremely Low
60	2	0.4	Extremely Low
55	1	0.1	Extremely Low

Percentiles are slightly different as these are ordinal data, which range from 0 to 100, and their values tell you what percentage of the standardisation sample scored at or below that level. For example, a percentile score (or rank) of 50 is the median, which means that half the population scored at or below this. A percentile score of over 98 would mean this is a score which only the top 2 percent of the population achieved. If scores are normally distributed, there will be a reliable correspondence between index scores, scaled scores, and percentiles. If not, this means the scores in the standardisation sample were not normally distributed. Table 4.2 gives examples of these relationships.

The index scores represent the bottom and mid-point of each classification range. Whilst the correspondence between standardised scores and percentiles will not vary, so long as scores are normally distributed the terms that are used to describe them may do. The system used here is that originally used with the Wechsler intelligence tests and memory scales (Wechsler, 2008b), and is used with other tests from the same publisher. Where the different categories start and finish is based around percentiles, with the average range being the middle 50%.

There are numerous other classification systems, some of which use the same category ranges but different nomenclature, whereas others base their category ranges around standard deviations. For example, the Kaufman Assessment Battery for Children (Kaufman et al., 2005) uses one standard deviation above and below the mean as the average range, which includes roughly 64% of the population. I do not advocate the use of one system over another, but caution that consistency is required in which system is used. You cannot describe the same score as being within the average range in one place, and within the high average range somewhere else. General convention is to capitalise the first letter of each term to identify when the Wechsler system is being used (i.e. 'High Average' rather than 'high average').

How to Tell If a Score Is Significant?

The use of the normal distribution and probability comes into play when determining whether an apparently low score is acceptable or an indicator of decline. It is important not to overinterpret small differences as some degree of variation in scores is not unusual – the question is how much? Traditionally, in measurement of many naturally occurring phenomena, the 5th and 2nd percentiles have been used as cut-offs for what was considered 'normal'.

Using the 5th percentile means that a score is lower than would be expected in 95% of people, and was used as a cut-off in the design of some cognitive tests (e.g. Warrington, 1996). The 2nd percentile represents roughly 2 standard deviations below the mean and has traditionally been taken to indicate impaired performance on a test (Cimino, 2000). For dementia diagnosis, DSM-V recommends using a cut-off of two or more standard deviations below 'appropriate norms' for major neurocognitive disorder (dementia), and 1–1.5 standard deviations for a diagnosis of mild neurocognitive disorder (MCI). The difficulty with this approach is that ability on a test is usually affected by factors such as age and educational level. Whilst most tests have norms for different age ranges, few have this further subdivided according to educational level; in fact, doing do would rapidly result in very small normative groups, or would require extremely large standardisation samples. The approach favoured by neuropsychologists has therefore been to derive an estimate of the person's premorbid ability.

Estimating Premorbid Ability

There have been a number of different methods proposed for this purpose, such as using the highest score achieved by a person, 'hold-tests' (those least sensitive to decline), and demographic variables (Lezak et al., 2012). The approach which has emerged as most widely used is based on the logic of the hold-test and consists of reading aloud a list of words with atypical spelling–sound correspondences, known as irregular words (Nelson & O'Connell, 1978; Wechsler, 2011). The rationale is that irregular words contain spelling–sound combinations other than those commonly found in the language. If attempting to read them aloud using general rules about spelling–sound correspondences, they will be mispronounced, resulting in a 'regularisation' error. You therefore need to be familiar with each word to some extent, and the number of such words you can read correctly correlates with your IQ.

This brings us to the third essential statistic mentioned earlier: the correlation. This describes the strength of a relationship between two variables – for example, the scores on a reading test such as the Test of Premorbid Function (TOPF) (Wechsler, 2011) and another test of ability such as the WAIS-IV (Wechsler, 2008b). Having established that there is an acceptable relationship between two variables, it is possible to use another correlation-based technique, 'linear regression', to use the score on the first variable to predict the score on the second variable. It is sometimes possible to add additional variables, which also have acceptable correlations, to increase the accuracy of predictions; this is known as 'multiple regression'.

Such tests are then used to estimate where someone's premorbid ability is likely to have fallen and consider the discrepancy between the estimated premorbid and current scores to determine if there is evidence of a deterioration. It should be noted that this is not an exact science, and the accuracy is reduced further if the test used to estimate premorbid ability has not been co-normed within the same sample as the test it is intended to predict. Unfortunately, standardising any test requires large sample sizes and considerable resources, which means that methods of estimating premorbid function are not standardised against many of the tests we might wish to use in a neuropsychological assessment.

A compromise approach is often adopted by many practitioners for estimating the person's full-scale IQ, with the assumption that other cognitive scores will fall within the same range. This method is prone to a degree of inaccuracy as specific cognitive abilities can differ considerably from the general ability factor which this approach seeks to estimate (Schinka & Vanderploeg, 2000).

Another method of estimating premorbid ability is based around the use of demographic variables such as age, years of education, and occupation (Crawford & Allan, 1997). This is often done in addition to a reading-based score to increase predictive power, or when a reading-based test is not appropriate. For example, if someone's language processing has been affected, if they have developmental dyslexia, or if they do not have English as a first language, a reading-based test may not be accurate. Reading-based tests are generally more accurate predictors within a non-impaired sample, but demographic variables have the advantage of being, by definition, premorbid. Using both together gives the greatest degree of accuracy (Crawford, Nelson et al., 1990; Crawford, Cochrane et al., 1990).

Base Rates

The concept of base rates in psychology can be traced back to at least the 1950s and an article by Meehl and Rosen (1955), although their use in neuropsychology became more common place with the introduction of WAIS-III (Wechsler, 1997a) and WMS-III (Wechsler, 1997b). Base rates refer to the frequency of occurrence within the standardisation sample – for example, the percentage of the sample which showed a difference of a certain size between two index scores, or between an obtained index score and an estimated premorbid score. A difference may be statistically significant (as in reliable), but still may not be a particularly rare occurrence. Although there is always a degree of arbitrariness when deciding on what cut-off to use for deciding between a normal and an abnormal discrepancy, a difference seen in less than 5% of the population would typically be considered abnormal.

A slightly different approach was advocated by Brooks, Iverson, Feldman, and Holdnack (2009) for considering the probability of achieving a low test score when considering individual subtests rather than index scores. They pointed out that occasional low scores are relatively common among healthy people, and the more tests administered, the greater the likelihood of achieving a low score. There are also factors relating to the individual, such as years of education, which influence how many low scores might be expected. For example, if administering WAIS-IV and WMS-IV to someone of Average ability, it would be possible to take the number of low subtest scores the person achieved (e.g. below the 5th percentile) and look up what percentage of the standardisation sample also achieved that number of low scores. If for example, 30% of the population in that ability range had 3 scores below the 5th percentile, that is not particularly unusual. If only 4% of the population had that number of low scores, it could be considered abnormal.

Whilst the logic behind this is immediately appealing, there are also some limitations. The first problem is that not all test batteries have base rates available. The second problem is that the probability of achieving a low score is directly related to the total number of subtests administered. If we imagine the WAIS-IV and WMS-IV are the assessments of choice, but the examiner decided to use shortened versions of each, the probability of a low score would change. Consequently, the use of base rates may not be as common as one might expect given the clear advantages associated with their use.

Evaluating Change

Memory clinics are one of the few contexts in which a neuropsychologist might be asked to assess a person more than once, often if the initial assessment did not indicate a deterioration in function, but the person has continued to experience a subjective decline. Presuming that the same tests are administered on both occasions, the question will arise of whether there has been a significant change in test scores? The most basic and simple way of addressing this is to consider whether the confidence intervals for the scores on the different administrations overlap. Confidence intervals are routinely calculated for the index scores on tests such as the WAIS-IV, WMS-S, and RBANS (Randolph et al., 1998), and tables are provided for looking up the values rather than calculating them. If there is no overlap, the difference is significant.

More sophisticated and complex methods have been devised over the years, the best known of which is the reliable change index (Jacobson, Follette, & Ravenstorf, 1984), originally devised for the purpose of evaluating outcomes in psychotherapy research. Although numerous variants have subsequently been developed, often with the intention of accounting for regression to the mean, Morely (2018) recommended using the original method as none of the more complex methods had any demonstrable superiority. Formulas for calculating confidence intervals and reliable change are included in the chapter appendix.

A further consideration when reassessing a patient is whether to readminister the original tests or to use a parallel battery. Whilst a parallel battery may intuitively appear to be a good idea, there are problems associated with this approach, the first being that few tests have parallel versions available. Also, in some instances the parallel versions may have been standardised on a smaller sample and have lower reliability scores compared to repeating the same test twice. However, in most cases where a parallel version of a test is available, it is considered a preferable option to readministering the same test.

It should be noted that there are very few parallel versions available of executive tests. This is because executive tests often incorporate a degree of novelty, and therefore show particularly poor test–retest reliability (Burgess, 2003). There are some exceptions to this, the most notable being verbal fluency, where different versions of the test have been normed using different letters.

Table 4.3 Aspects of cognitive function to cover as part of a neuropsychological assessment

Aspect of cognitive function	Examples of disorders where an early decline in this aspect of function may be seen
Speed of Information Processing	Vascular dementia, subcortical dementias
Attention	Vascular dementia, Parkinson's disease
Memory	Alzheimer's disease
Perception	Posterior cortical atrophy
Language	Primary progressive aphasia
Executive Function	Behavioural variant frontotemporal dementia

What Should Be Covered in a Neuropsychological Assessment for Dementia?

Having stated that some quantitative estimate of premorbid ability should be included, the question arises of which aspects of cognition to cover. There is not complete consistency regarding the fundamental aspects of cognition, but the areas outlined in Table 4.3 are suggested as selective deficits in each of these may point towards a differential diagnosis. These are organised so that the first letters spell the word SAMPLE, which can be used as mnemonic to help remember what to cover. Further detail can be found in the chapters on specific types of dementia.

In addition to these areas – and, of course, qualitative information – a quantitative measure of mood, such as an inventory, may be useful.

Test Selection

In the context of a memory clinic with many frail and elderly patients, the standard protocol of 'use the tests with the best psychometric properties' is not always easy to follow. If we wish to use a set of tests which are co-normed on a large population, and which allow us to make use of extensive psychometric data for comparisons including base rates, few (if any) tests can compete with the combination of WAIS-IV, WMS-IV, and TOPF (Wechsler 2008a, 2008b, 2011). Whilst these tests are extensive, they do not cover all aspects of cognition, so additional tests would need to be added to assess executive function. Should there be possible concerns regarding visuospatial processing and language, further tests might also be incorporated to address these areas. Whilst this would undoubtedly result in a very comprehensive assessment, it may also take up to four hours to complete. This is unlikely to be possible in many healthcare services, and there is also the question of how lengthy an assessment a patient may tolerate before it impacts upon their performance. On the other hand, the neuropsychological assessment must be able to generate more extensive information than can be ascertained from a screening instrument. It is therefore usually a question of using tests which give the most amount of information whilst working within operational and clinical constraints. If you only have two hours for each assessment, including taking a history, a far briefer core assessment, such as the Repeatable Battery for the Assessment of Neuropsychological Function (RBANS, Randolph et al., 1998) may be more appropriate.

Performance Validity

When considering any form of assessment, the concepts of reliability and validity must be taken into account. Reliability refers to the extent to which tests give consistent results, and validity refers to whether tests measure what they purport to measure. A major area of research in neuropsychology has been the area of performance validity testing (previously referred to as effort testing), which aims to identity whether a set of test results are likely to be a true/valid representation of a person's cognitive ability. The phrase 'non-credible performance' has gained popularity to describe a set of results which are unlikely to be valid, as this refrains from implying an explanation for the apparent lack of validity.

Various methods have been devised for identifying possible invalid test profiles, and these can be divided into stand-alone measures and embedded measures. The former are tests designed specifically for this purpose and are administered in addition to a battery of cognitive tests. These include the Test of Memory Malingering (TOMM) (Tombaugh, 1996), the Word Memory Test (WMT) (Green, 2003), and the Medical Symptom Validity Test (MSVT) (Green, 2004). Embedded measures are scores, or algorithms, derived from existing test batteries, such as the Reliable Digit Span (Greiffenstein, Baker, and Gola, 1994) and the Effort Scale (ES; Novitski et al., 2012) based on the RBANS Randolph et al., 1998). A further distinction is made between symptom validity tests, which are based on self-reported symptoms, and performance validity tests (PVTs), which are designed to identify non-credible performance on objective tests of cognition (Larrabee, 2012). Although the use of PVTs is recommended by both the British Psychological Society (McMillan et al., 2009) and the American Academy of Clinical Neuropsychology (Heilbronner et al., 2009), surveys of neuropsychologist practice in the UK have suggested this is not done routinely in many areas of assessment (Lenherr & Gerhand, 2012; McCarter et al., 2009).

The assessment of mild cognitive impairment and dementia may be a particularly tricky area as research has shown that a significant number of patients score below cut-off on PVTs. For example, performance on the TOMM (Tombaugh, 1996) has been reported to be robust in MCI, but less so in patients with dementia (Teichner & Wagner, 2004; Walter et al., 2014). Dean et al. (2009) looked at 18 PVTs in a sample of 214 patients with dementia. The majority of tests showed specificity scores within the range of 30–70%, although recommended cut-offs for digit span indicators showed a specificity of 90%. Rudman et al. (2011) looked at a range of PVTs in a sample of patients with young-onset dementia, and found that only the Rey's Dot Counting Test was passed by everybody.

McGuire, Crawford and Evans (2017) reviewed the literature on PVTs in dementia and recommended the use of tests which employ a hierarchical approach by incorporating a profile analysis. For example, the WMT (Green, 2003), the MSVT (Green, 2004) and the non-verbal MSVT (Green, 2008) begin by using a PVT with a cut-off score. However, the participants then proceed to complete several other subtests which are conventional memory subtests. The performance on the PVT subtests is compared to the performance on the conventional memory subtests, with scrutiny of the difference between these different sets of scores. Patients with dementia show a large difference, whereas controls requested to feign impairment do not. This was referred to as a dementia profile. Green, Montijo, and Brockhaus (2011) reported that 63% of patients with dementia and 21.6% of MCI patients failed the PVTs, but all of their dementia group exhibited the dementia profile. It should be noted, however, that completing the full versions of these tests, including the conventional memory subtests, is more time-consuming and may not be practical when there is limited time available for an assessment.

Using similar logic, Gerhand, Hacker, and Jones (2021) advocated the interpretation of PVTs with an emphasis on context and consistency. For example, when PVT scores fall below cut-off in an assessment, there should be consideration of whether there may be an incentive to underperform, as outlined in Sherman, Slick, and Iverserson's (2020) revised criteria for malingering. In addition to this, when determining if below-cut-off scores may result from genuine cognitive difficulties, questions should be asked to ascertain whether this interpretation is consistent with:

- Performance on other tests (e.g. do they do reasonably well on hard tests while performing badly on easier tests?)
- The person's everyday function (e.g. do they show very low cognitive scores whilst performing at a reasonably high level in everyday life?)
- A known organic disorder (e.g. does the test profile make sense in the context of other aspects of their presentation?)

Context and consistency is always of primary importance when interpreting any neuropsychological data.

Key Points

- A neuropsychological assessment is most useful when there is uncertainty regarding whether there has been a decline in cognition from a previous level.
- Some knowledge of psychometrics is required to undertake and interpret a neuropsychological assessment. Key statistical concepts to understand are the mean, the standard deviation, and the correlation. Many more complex concepts take these as their starting point.
- A number of different standardised scores are used in neuropsychology. It is important to understand the relationship between these scores, and how they translate into percentiles.
- A big advantage of neuropsychological assessment over a screening instrument is the ability to estimate premorbid ability. This allows a more accurate appraisal of whether any low cognitive scores represent decline from a previous level.
- Performance validity should be considered in any assessment; however, most PVTs can be failed by people with dementia. Whether a cognitive profile is valid should always be evaluated by considering context and the consistency.
- Whilst test selection generally prioritises psychometric properties, when working with clients who may be frail, covering the full range of cognitive abilities in the least number of tests may have to be considered.

Appendix D Formulas and Calculations

The Mean

The mean is the average value and is calculated by adding up all of the scores and dividing this figure by the number of scores.

The standard deviation is a representation of how spread out scores are around the mean. It is calculated as follows:

1. Subtract each score from the mean
2. Square each value, which removes any negative values
3. Calculate the sum of these values
4. Divide the total by the number of scores
5. Take the square root of this number

The Confidence Interval

A lot of test manuals provide you with confidence intervals for scores. There are also a number of websites which allow you to just key in values and have the confidence interval calculated for you. It is quite unlikely that you will need to calculate a confidence interval by hand, but in case that happens, here is an explanation of how to do it.

As you might imagine from reading this chapter, it starts with the mean and standard deviation. In this instance, the mean is the score of interest. You also need the number of observations (i.e. sample size) and the z score of the number for which you wish to calculate a confidence interval. For a 95% confidence interval you use a z score of 1.96. You then use the following formula:

The score of interest $+/- 1.96 \times [\text{standard deviation}/n]$

If you wish to know whether there is a significant difference between two scores, the simplest way to determine this is to see if the confidence intervals overlap or not. If they do not overlap, the difference is significant.

Reliable Change Index

This is a method for calculating whether there is a significant difference between test scores taken on two different occasions, taking into account the reliability of the test. The following method, based on Jacobsen & Truax (1991), is calculated by dividing the change in the person's score by the standard error of the difference for the test.

As you might expect, the starting point is the standard deviation, from which we calculate the standard error of measurement:

$\text{SEM} = s\sqrt{1 - rxx}$

SD is the standard deviation and R is the reliability figure for the test, either based on test–retest or Cronbach's alpha.

The standard error of the difference is calculated as follows:

$\text{SDIFF} = \sqrt{2(\text{SEM}^2)}$

The reliable change is the difference between the two scores divided by the standard error of the difference. To be reliable, this figure needs to be greater than or equal to 1.96.

References

Brooks, B. L., Iverson, G. L., Feldman, H. H., & Holdnack, J. A. (2009). Minimizing misdiagnosis: Psychometric criteria for possible or probable memory impairment. *Dementia and Geriatric Cognitive Disorders*, 27, 439–50.

Burgess, P., & Shallice, T. (1997). *The Hayling and Brixton Tests: Test Manual*. Bury St. Edmunds: Thames Valley Test Company.

Burgess, P. (2003). Assessment of executive function. In P. W. Halligan, U. Kischka & J. C Marshall (Eds.), *Handbook of Clinical Neuropsychology*. Oxford, Oxford University Press.

Cimino, C. R. (2000). Principles of neuropsychological interpretation. In R. D. Vanderploeg (Ed.), *Clinician's Guide to Neuropsychological Assessment*, 2nd ed. London: Lawrence Erlbaum Associates.

Crawford, J. R., & Allan, K. M. (1997). Estimating premorbid WAIS-R IQ with demographic variables: Regression equations derived from a UK sample. *The Clinical Neuropsychologist*, 11(2), 192–7.

Crawford, J. R., Cochrane, R. H. B., Besson, J. A. O., Parker, D. M., & Stewart, L. E. (1990). Premorbid IQ estimates obtained by combining the NART and demographic variables: Construct validity. *Personality and Individual Differences*, 11(2), 209–10.

Crawford, J. R., Nelson, H. E., Blackmore, L., Cochrane, R. H. B., & Allan, K. M. (1990). Estimating premorbid intelligence by combining the NART and demographic variables: An examination of the NART standardisation sample and supplementary equations. *Personality and Individual Differences*, 11(11), 1153–7.

Dean, A., Victor, T., Boone, K., Philpott, L., & Hess, R. (2009) Dementia and effort test performance. *The Clinical Neuropsychologist*, 23(1), 133–52.

Ellis, A. W., & Young, A. W. (1988). *Human Cognitive Neuropsychology*. London: Psychology Press.

Fodor, J. (1983). *The Modularity of Mind*. Cambridge, MA. MIT Press.

Gerhand, S., Jones, C. A., & Hacker, D. (2021). Effort testing, performance validity, and the importance of context and consistency. In P. S. Moore, S. Brifcani, & A. Worthington (Eds.), *Neuropsychological Aspects of Brain Injury Litigation* (pp. 89–115). London: Routledge.

Green, P. (2003). *Word Memory Test for Windows: User's Manual and Program*. Edmonton: Green's Publishing.

Green, P. (2004). *Manual for the Medical Symptom Validity Test*. Edmonton: Green's Publishing.

Green, P. (2008). *Test Manual for the Nonverbal Medical Symptom Validity Test*. Edmonton: Green's Publishing.

Green, P., Montijo, J., & Brockhaus, R. (2011). High specificity of the word memory test and medical symptom validity test in groups with severe verbal memory impairment. *Applied Neuropsychology*, 18, 86–94.

Greiffenstein, M. F., Baker, W. J., & Gola, T. (1994). Validation of malingered amnesia measures with a large clinical sample. *Psychological Assessment*, 6, 218–24.

Heilbronner, R. L., Sweet, J. J., Morgan, J. E., et al. (2009). American Academy of Clinical Neuropsychology consensus conference statement on the neuropsychological assessment of effort, response bias, and malingering. *The Clinical Neuropsychologist*, 23, 1093–129.

Jacobson, N. S., & Truax, P. (1991). Clinical significance: A statistical approach to defining meaningful change in psychotherapy research. *Journal of Consulting & Clinical Psychology*, 59, 12–19.

Jacobson, N. S., Follett, W. C., & Revenstorf, D. (1984). Psychotherapy outcome research – methods for reporting variability and evaluating clinical significance. *Behavior Therapy*, 15(4), 336–52.

Kaufman, A. S., Lichtenberger, E., Fletcher-Janzen, E., & Kaufman, N. L. (2005). *Essentials of KABC-II Assessment*. Hoboken: Wiley.

Larrabee, G. J. (2012). Performance validity and symptom validity in neuropsychological assessment. *Journal of the International Neuropsychological Society*, **18**(4), 625–31.

Lenherr, S., & Gerhand, S. (2012). A survey of neuropsychological test use among DON members. *British Psychological Society, Division of Neuropsychology Newsletter*, **11**(2), 9–12.

Lezak, M., Howieson, D., Bigler, E., & Tranel, D. (2012). *Neuropsychological Assessment* (4th ed.). Oxford: Oxford University Press.

McCarter, R. J., Walton, N. H., Brooks, D. N., & Powell, G. E. (2009). Effort testing in contemporary UK neuropsychological practice. *The Clinical Neuropsychologist*, **23**, 1050–66.

McGuire, C., Crawford, S., & Evans, J. J. (2017). Effort testing in dementia assessment: A systematic review. *Archives of Clinical Neuropsychology*, **34**, 114–31.

McMillan, T. M., Anderson, S., Baker, G., et al. (2009). *Assessment of Effort in Clinical Testing of Cognitive Functioning for Adults*. Leicester: British Psychological Society.

Meehl, P. E., & Rosen, A. (1955) Antecedent probability and the efficiency of psychometric signs, patterns, or cutting scores. *Psychological Bulletin*, **52**, 194–216.

Morley, S. (2018). *Single Case Methods in Clinical Psychology: A Practical Guide*. New York: Routledge.

Nelson, H. E., & O'Connell, A. (1978). Dementia: The estimation of premorbid intelligence levels using the New Adult Reading Test. *Cortex*, **14**(2), 234–44.

Novitski, J., Steele, S., Karantzoulis, S., & Randolph, C. (2012). The repeatable battery for the assessment of neuropsychological status effort scale. *Archives of Clinical Neuropsychology*, **27**, 190–5.

Plaut, D. (1995). Double dissociation without modularity: Evidence from connectionist neuropsychology *Journal of Clinical and Experimental Neuropsychology*, **17**(2), 291–321.

Randolph, C., Tierney, M. C., Mohr, E., & Chase, T. N. (1998). The repeatable battery for the assessment of neuropsychological status (RBANS): Preliminary clinical validity. *Journal*

of *Clinical & Experimental Neuropsychology*, **20**, 310–19.

Rudman, N., Oyebode, J., Jones, C., & Bentham, P. (2011). An investigation into the validity of effort tests in a working age dementia population. *Aging and Mental Health*, **15**(1), 47–57.

Schinka, J. A., & Vanderpoeg, R. D. (2000). Estimating premorbid level of functioning. In R. D. Vanderploeg (Ed.), *Clinician's Guide to Neuropsychological Assessment* (2nd Ed.). London: Lawrence Earlbaum Associates.

Sherman, E., Slick, D., & Iversen, G. (2020). Multidimensional Malingering Criteria for neuropsychological assessment: A 20-year update of the Malingered Neuropsychological Dysfunction Criteria. *Journal of Clinical and Experimental Neuropsychology*, **35**(6), 735–64.

Teichner, G., & Wagner, M. T. (2004). The Test of Memory Malingering (TOMM): Normative data from cognitively intact, cognitively impaired, and elderly patients with dementia. *Archives of Clinical Neuropsychology*, **19**(3), 455–64.

Tombaugh, T. N. (1996). *The Test of Memory Malingering*. Toronto: MultiHealth Systems.

Walter, J., Morris, J., Swier-Vosnos, A., & Pliskin, N. (2014). Effects of severity of dementia on a symptom validity measure. *The Clinical Neuropsychologist*, **28**(7), 1197–208.

Warrington, E. (1996). *The Camden Memory Tests – Manual*. Hove: Psychology Press.

Wechsler, D. (1997a). *WAIS-III administration and scoring manual*. San Antonio: Psychological Corporation.

Wechsler, D. (1997b). *Wechsler Adult Intelligence Scale – III*. New York: Psychological Corporation.

Wechsler, D. (2008a). *Wechsler Adult Intelligence Scale* (4th ed.). *Technical and Interpretive Manual*. San Antonia: NCS Pearson Inc.

Wechsler, D. (2008b). *Wechsler Memory Scale* (4th ed.). San Antonia: Pearson.

Wechsler, D. (2011). *Test of Premorbid Functioning. UK version (TOPF UK)*. London: Pearson Assessment.

Alzheimer's Disease

Dementia of the Alzheimer's Type (DAT) is known to present in a number of different forms. This chapter will first consider the most common, 'typical' variant, before considering the less common, atypical variants. The chapter will also include a summary of limbic-predominant age-related TDP-43 encephalopathy (LATE) (Dickson et al., 1994; Nelson et al., 2019), a recently identified degenerative disorder affecting older adults which closely resembles DAT in its clinical presentation.

Whilst diagnosis of DAT is likely to be transformed by the use of biomarkers, at the time of writing these are not widely available in most healthcare settings, and diagnosis is based upon clinical presentation.

Prevalence and Incidence

DAT accounts for up to 60–80% of cases (Alzheimer Association, 2022). Although DAT is commonly accepted as the most common cause of dementia, evidence from recent post-mortem studies suggests that more than 50% of cases of DAT occur with comorbidities, such as vascular dementia (VD) and dementia with Lewy bodies (DLB) (Brenowitz et al., 2017; Kapasi, DeCarli, & Schneider, 2017). This is referred to as 'mixed dementia'. As the incidence of both DAT and VD increase with age, it is perhaps unsurprising that mixed dementia is most common in adults aged over 85 (De Reuck et al., 2018; James et al., 2017). TDP-43 and hippocampal sclerosis are also pathologies which can co-occur with DAT, and the presence of multiple pathologies is likely to lower the threshold for developing dementia (Kapasi et al., 2017).

The prevalence of DAT has consistently been shown to increase with age. In a metanalysis of prevalence rates in Europe, Niu et al. (2017) reported the following prevalence rates for different age ranges, displayed in Table 5.1.

A similar pattern of increase with age has been reported for prevalence rates in America (based on the 2020 US census), although with slightly higher figures for each age range (Rajan et al., 2021), displayed in Table 5.2.

Most studies show a higher prevalence rate in women, with two-thirds of people with DAT in America being female (Alzheimer Association, 2022), which has traditionally been attributed to women living longer. Other explanations have also been put forward, such as hormonal differences and the effect of menopause (Tang et al., 1996). Hormone replacement therapy has been associated with a reducing risk of developing DAT by 11–33% (Stute et al., 2021). However, Wu et al. (2020) suggested this is only the case for the first five years of treatment and may actually increase the risk thereafter. There has also been evidence for a difference between surgical and natural menopause, with the latter not

Table 5.1 European prevalence rates for Alzheimer's Disease in different age ranges

Age range in years	Prevalence
65–74	0.97%
75–84	7.66%
85+	22.53%

Table 5.2 North American prevalence rates for Alzheimer's Disease in different age ranges

Age range in years	Prevalence
65–74	5.0%
75–84	13.1%
85+	33.2%

Table 5.3 European incidence rates for Alzheimer's Disease in different age ranges

Age range in years	Incidence
65–74	4.43 per thousand person years
75–84	13.78 per thousand person years
85+	35.74 per thousand person years

Table 5.4 European incidence rates for Alzheimer's Disease in different age ranges

Age range in years	Incidence
65–74	4 per thousand person years
75–84	32 per thousand person years
85+	76 per thousand person years

showing an association with cognitive decline (Henderson & Sherwin, 2007). The age at which surgical menopause occurs may also be a factor, with earlier age of menopause being associated with increased DAT pathology (Bove et al., 2014).

Nui et al. (2017) reported the following incidence rates for Europe, displayed in Table 5.3. The 2010 US census reported the following incidence rates (Rajan et al., 2019) (Table 5.4).

Gao et al. (2019) looked at the change in incidence rates over time and reported that while incidence rates for dementia as a whole had decreased, incidence rates for DAT had remained stable.

Although the biggest single risk factor for developing DAT is advancing age, roughly 10% of cases occur before the age of 65, referred to as young-onset Alzheimer's disease (YOAD). This has been associated with a more rapid rate of decline, although this has not been demonstrated in all studies (Stanley & Walker, 2014). Autosomal dominant familial DAT is more common in YOAD, while the typical sporadic form of the disease seen in late-onset Alzheimer's disease (LOAD) is rare in individuals under 50 (Rossor et al., 2010). Psychiatric symptoms are more frequently reported in YOAD, with depression being more common in females and anxiety presenting more often in males (Gumus et al., 2021). Atypical variants of DAT are also more commonly found in YOAD (Koedam et al., 2010), accounting for roughly 25% of cases (van der Flier et al., 2011). While YOAD has traditionally been considered a purer form of the disease, Spina et al. (2021) found non-Alzheimer neuropathology to be relatively common in a consecutive autopsy study. Although the overall rate and number of comorbidities was higher in their LOAD sample, they still found evidence of at least one non-Alzheimer neuropathology in 98% of their YOAD group. Lewy bodies and cerebral amyloid angiopathy were common in both groups.

Time Course and the DAT Continuum

The vast majority of cases of DAT develop slowly over many years, with evidence that pathological changes may begin more than 20 years before the development of symptoms (Braak et al., 2011). Following diagnosis, the life expectancy of someone for typical DAT with onset over 65 is 4–8 years (Alzheimer Association, 2022), although some cases can exceed this. Life expectancy typically decreases the older the person is at diagnosis (Tom et al., 2015).

A continuum has been proposed describing the progression of DAT (Aisen et al., 2017) which may standardise the terminology used to describe the different stages as the literature on DAT has sometimes used different terms to describe the same thing (e.g. prodromal, preclinical, and MCI). This necessitates the use of biomarkers to confirm the presence of underlying Alzheimer-type pathology, which, as mentioned earlier, are not commonly available in clinical practice at the time of writing. The continuum, which is presented in Table 5.5, is covered here on the assumption that this situation may change within a reasonable timescale. It is perhaps worth restating that dementia is a syndrome, for which Alzheimer's disease can be a possible cause, and it is possible to have Alzheimer's disease without having dementia.

Pathology

The pathological changes associated with DAT have been extensively studied, beginning with the post-mortem identification of abnormal cells in the very first patient studied by Alois Alzheimer in 1907. There are two types of abnormal cell, which have been named senile plaques and neurofibrillary tangles, and they are associated with different types of abnormal protein. Plaques occur outside the cells, and are formed from beta amyloid protein (Glenner et al., 1984), whereas tangles occur within the cells and are formed from phosphorylated tau protein (Brion et al., 1985). Tau is associated with a number of different neurodegenerative disorders, whereas beta amyloid is specific to Alzheimer's. The presence of both proteins is required for a biological (as opposed to a purely clinical) diagnosis (Jack et al., 2018). There is a reliable progression of pathology in the typical form of Alzheimer's, which develops as follows: medial temporal lobes around the entorhinal region, and

Table 5.5 A proposed continuum to describe the progression of DAT (Aisen et al., 2017)

Stage	Characteristics
Preclinical	Evidence of Alzheimer-type pathology, identified by the use of biomarkers, not accompanied by a decline in cognition or any other identifiable symptoms
Mild cognitive impairment	Measurable evidence of cognitive decline, with memory 1–1.5 standard deviations lower than expected. Still able to function on a daily basis, albeit with more effort/errors
Mild Alzheimer's dementia	Evidence of two or more aspects of cognitive function falling more than 2 standard deviations lower than expected Difficulty with some aspect of *instrumental* activities of daily living, to the extent they can no longer be performed without assistance
Moderate Alzheimer's dementia	Evidence of two or more aspects of cognitive function falling more than 2 standard deviations lower than expected. Difficulty with some aspect of *basic* activities of daily living, to the extent they can no longer be performed without assistance
Severe Alzheimer's dementia	As above, but with a requirement for support with almost all activities of daily living

spreading out to limbic areas → higher-order processing areas of basal temporal lobe, basal frontal, and occipital areas → sensory areas affected last (Braak & Braak, 1996). This progression is reflected in the development of atrophy, which is initially most pronounced in the temporal lobes and the medial parietal cortex but becomes more widespread as the disease progresses (Fox & Schott, 2004). Annual rates of global brain atrophy have been reported to be 2% in Alzheimer's disease compared with 0.4% in healthy age-matched controls (Silbert et al., 2003).

Research into Alzheimer's began to accelerate following the identification of the proteins associated with plaques as beta amyloid (Glenner et al., 1984) and with tangles as tau (Brion et al., 1985). Hardy and Higgins (1992) put forward the 'amyloid cascade hypothesis', which considered an imbalance between the production and clearance of beta amyloid protein to be key in the development of DAT. Beta amyloid builds up, causing inflammation, oxidation, and neuronal loss, which in turn accelerates the accumulation of the phosphorylated tau protein that makes up the neurofibrillary tangles. This theory has been highly influential, although it has been suggested that this on its own may not be sufficient to give a full explanation of how DAT develops (Herrup, 2015). The development of biomarkers such as amyloid PET scans has shown that 20–30% of older adults without signs of cognitive decline have an accumulation of beta amyloid protein (Jack et al., 2014), and clinical trials in humans using drugs to remove beta amyloid have not been successful in achieving clinical improvement (Vellas et al., 2013) (although see Chapter 11).

Tau protein accumulates within the cell body of neurons, eventually enveloping the entire cell, causing cell death (Maccioni et al., 2010). Tau protein is associated with several dementias which do not feature prominent beta amyloid accumulation. It is also found in the brains of healthy older adults without evidence of cognitive decline (Bennett et al., 2006). The build-up in DAT appears to begin in the medial temporal lobe, but there is evidence that it does not spread beyond this area unless beta amyloid is also present (Price & Morris, 1999; Schöll et al., 2016). At present, the nature of the relationship between beta amyloid and tau protein in the development of DAT remains unclear.

Genetics

A genetic link is most commonly seen in YOAD, with 35–60% of patients having at least one first-degree relative affected and 10–15% of familial cases being autosomal dominant (i.e. inherited from one parent) (Cacace, Sleegers, & Van Broeckhoven, 2016). Three relevant genes were identified as APP, coding for amyloid precursor protein, PSEN1 coding for presenilin 1, and PSEN2 coding for presenilin 2. However, these genes are found in a relatively small number of families, and not at all in cases of LOAD, which is considered to be mainly sporadic.

With LOAD, a number of genes have been identified as possible risk factors, with the most well-known being the APOE-E gene (Saunders et al., 1993), which has the strongest genetic link. A variant of this gene (ε4) increases the likelihood of developing DAT. Approximately 25% of the population have one copy of APOE-ε4, which doubles the risk of developing Alzheimer's disease (Alzheimer's Society, 2020). Inheriting this gene confers a fivefold greater risk of developing the disease, but still does not mean everyone with this gene will develop DAT (Alzheimer's Society, 2020), as non-genetic factors also play a role. International consortiums of genome-wide association studies have identified more than 40 genes which are thought to have some association with Alzheimer's disease, although the extent to which there is a causal link has yet to be confirmed (Bellenguez, Grenier-Boley, & Lambert, 2020).

Diagnostic Criteria

At present we are going through a transition period for diagnostic criteria as a result of successful development of biomarkers, which has led to the proposal of purely biological diagnostic criteria. These are currently aimed at research rather than clinical practice. Outlined by Jack et al. (2018), this is called the ATN system and uses biomarkers to detect the presence of beta amyloid protein (A), pathologic tau (T), and neurodegeneration (N). It also incorporates the continuum view of DAT as described earlier (Aisen et al., 2017). The presence of biomarkers identifying both beta amyloid and tau are required for a diagnosis of Alzheimer's disease, and where someone sits on the continuum is based on evidence of neurodegeneration and cognitive symptoms. It is argued that a biological approach is required as there are atypical presentations of Alzheimer's disease, and 10–30% of people clinically diagnosed with DAT are found at autopsy not to have Alzheimer-related pathological changes (Nelson et al., 2011). It also allows for those who may have Alzheimer-type pathology but are either cognitively normal or meet the criteria for MCI.

Whilst there are recommendations for how to incorporate the use of biomarkers into clinical diagnoses (Dubois et al., 2021), it is uncertain when they will become widely available. Consequently, the syndrome-based approach to diagnosis is likely to remain in place for clinical diagnosis for some time yet. The most widely used criteria for diagnosis of DAT are those put forward by the National Institute on Aging and the Alzheimer's Association (McKhann et al., 2011), which were a revision of earlier criteria put forward by the National Institute of Neurological and Communicative Disorders and Stroke and the Alzheimer's Disease and Related Disorders Association, known as the NINCDS-ADRDA criteria (McKhann et al., 1984). They align with the DSM-5 criteria for Major or Mild Neurocognitive Disorder Due to Alzheimer's Disease (American Psychiatric Association, 2013).

The criteria for dementia should first be met, before considering the subtype. There are two clinical categories of Probable and Possible DAT. *Probable* DAT with a typical presentation requires the following:

- Insidious onset over a period of months or years. DSM-5 also specifies there must be no extended plateaus
- Reported or observed history of worsening cognition
- Impaired learning and recall of recently learned information and evidence of dysfunction in at least one other cognitive domain
- DSM-5 has the additional criteria of no evidence of mixed aetiology, the presence of which would indicate a mixed dementia.

Atypical presentations are referred to as non-amnestic and require the following most prominent deficits, along with deficits in other cognitive domains:

- Language presentation: prominent deficits are in word-finding
- Visuospatial presentation: spatial cognition, including object agnosia, impaired face recognition, simultanagnosia, and alexia
- Executive dysfunction: reasoning, judgement, and problem solving

Exclusion criteria are:
- Substantial accompanying cerebrovascular disease
- Core features of DLB
- Prominent features of frontotemporal dementia, either behavioural variant, semantic dementia, or agrammatic primary progressive aphasia
- Evidence for another concurrent, active neurological disease/non-neurological medical comorbidity/medication known to produce a substantial dampening of cognitive ability

There is increased certainty with a documented cognitive decline or evidence of one of the three genetic mutations: APP, presenilin 1, and presenilin 2. The APOE gene was not included.

A diagnosis of *possible* DAT is made when the core features are met, but there is (1) a sudden onset or a lack of evidence of progressive cognitive decline or (2) evidence of a mixed presentation (e.g. vascular, DLB, neurological disease).

The introduction of biomarkers could lead to 'pathophysiologically proved' DAT if the core features are met and there is evidence of DAT pathology. A diagnosis of DAT would not be made if there is sufficient evidence for an alternative diagnosis or the AD biomarkers are negative.

Neuropsychological Assessment

Whilst some dementias have key diagnostic features which are not purely cognitive (e.g. hallucinations, fluctuations, and Parkinsonism in DLB, behavioural changes in frontotemporal dementia (FTD)), DAT primarily presents with changes in cognitive ability. With all focal presentations, the initial presenting cognitive difficulty guides diagnosis, so assessment in the early stages of the disease is likely to be the most informative. As the disease progresses, other aspects of cognitive function begin to decline, but the original cognitive impairment usually remains more severe in relative terms. A stage will ultimately be reached when all abilities measured fall within the impaired range, at which point cognitive assessment will no longer be informative for differential diagnosis.

There is an extensive literature documenting cognitive impairment in DAT, with a consensus that memory difficulties are usually the initial presenting problem. Anterograde amnesia (difficulty learning new information) is usually the initial complaint, and then some retrograde amnesia which is temporally graded – that is, good recall of more distant information and events, with poorer recall of recent information and events. Memory deficits are seen in other forms of dementia, but the key difference is they are not normally the earliest presenting feature, or are not as severe as that seen in DAT. Zakzanis, Leach, and Kaplan (1999) performed meta-analyses on papers describing cognitive deficits in various forms of dementia. In their review of 199 studies of cognitive testing for DAT, they reported the following deficits, ranging from most to least severe:

1. Delayed recall
2. Memory acquisition (immediate memory)
3. Language skills
4. Visuospatial, visuoperceptual, and constructional ability
5. Executive function (cognitive flexibility and abstraction)
6. Attention
7. Manual dexterity

They pointed out that the first four of these corresponded with the order in which Cummings and Benson (1992) noted the cognitive deficits in DAT to evolve.

Most Sensitive Tests for Alzheimer's Disease

Bäckman et al. (2005) carried out a meta-analysis on cognitive impairment in preclinical DAT (MCI), and reported that the largest memory impairments were seen for tasks with a delayed memory component, consistent with the meta-analysis by Zakanis et al. (1999) on clinical DAT. They concluded that transferring information from temporary storage to a more permanent representation is a hallmark of the memory deficit seen in DAT. Their analysis also indicated that verbal memory was more affected than visual memory, a finding which was also reported in previous studies (Arnaiz and Almkvist, 2003; Carlesimo & Oscar-Berman, 1992).

List learning tests, such as the Rey Auditory Learning test (Schmidt, 1996) and the California Verbal Learning test (Delis, Kramer, Kaplan, & Ober, 2000), have been shown to have high sensitivity to the memory deficits seen in early DAT (Rabin et al., 2009). Paired associate learning (PAL) in both verbal (Duchek, Cheney, & Ferraro, 1991) and visually presented mediums (Hicks et al., 2021) also has a high sensitivity. Story recall is a bit more problematic, as healthy older adults have sometimes been shown to demonstrate deficits (Johnson, Storandt, & Balota, 2003), and there has been some suggestion that story recall is more sensitive to executive deficits (Tremont et al., 2000).

Tests of verbal fluency have shown a reliable difference between performance on letter fluency and semantic fluency, with a greater deficit on tests of semantic fluency (Henry,

Crawford, & Phillips, 2004). This is likely because letter fluency is more dependent on executive processing (frontal lobes) whereas semantic fluency is more closely related to semantic memory (temporal lobes). Although confrontation naming deficits are widely reported, these may be more apparent as the disease progresses (Enwefa & Enwefa, 2018). Differences have been shown when comparing DAT to patients with VD, with more naming errors seen in DAT (Lukatela et al., 1998).

Executive function tends to decline as the disease progresses, and can be detected on a range of common tests of executive function. A degree of caution should be exercised when using tests reliant on colour perception, such as variants of the Stroop test (Stroop, 1935), as there is evidence for a deficit in colour processing which appears to be unrelated to the stage of the illness (Pache et al., 2003).

Atypical Presentations

A comprehensive review of atypical presentations is beyond the scope of this book. Here we present summaries of the three most common types of atypical presentations of DAT. All atypical presentations tend to be relatively early onset.

Posterior Cortical Atrophy

Posterior Cortical Atrophy (PCA) is most commonly an atypical variant of DAT, although PCA has also been reported with DLB pathology (Schott & Crutch, 2019) and corticobasal degeneration (Tang-Wai et al., 2003). Average age of onset has been reported as 58.9 years, with a typical age range from 50 to 65 (Schott & Crutch, 2019), and prevalence has been reported as 13% of early-onset dementias (Kodam et al., 2010). Post-mortem studies have found the distribution of beta amyloid protein to be similar to that of typical DAT, but there is a concentration of tau protein in the primary and secondary visual processing areas (Hof et al., 1997; Tang-Wai et al., 2003). Imaging studies are likely to show atrophy or hypometabolism in the occipital and parietal lobes.

Patients typically present with visual problems, such as difficulty parking their cars, and usually progress to difficulties with reading (Mendez, Ghajarania, & Perryman, 2002). They may experience problems locating objects in front of them in the presence of other items (simultanagnosia) and difficulty with face recognition (prosopagnosia) (Shott & Crutch, 2019). If there is involvement of the parietal lobe, control of voluntary movement (dyspraxia) can also be affected (McMonagal et al., 2006) – for example, when doing up a necktie, or buttoning a shirt. As a result of the primary visual nature of early symptoms, many cases are first seen by ophthalmology/optometry, where visual acuity is typically found to be normal and the illness may not initially be identified as a degenerative brain disorder. Most patients do not fit the commonly used criteria for dementia.

PCA is more likely to be identified by cognitive screening than by detailed neuropsychological assessment. For example, impairment may be observed on clock drawing, figure copy, calculation, and spelling on instruments such as the ACE-III (Schott & Crutch, 2019). Difficulty may also be apparent in object recognition tasks such as fragmented letters. Detailed diagnostic criteria were published by Crutch et al. (2017), which state exclusion criteria are difficulties with anterograde memory, speech and language, executive function, and personality.

Logopenic Variant Primary Progressive Aphasia

Primary progressive aphasia (PPA) is more common as a form of FTD, with the original two subtypes being agrammatic and semantic dementia (Mesulam et al., 2012). However, a third type exists which is associated (although not exclusively) with DAT pathology (Gorno-Tempini et al., 2004). The easiest way to conceptualise PPA is in terms of how it relates to classic aphasia syndromes (Marshall et al., 2018), with logopenic variant primary progressive apahsia (lvPPA) corresponding loosely to conduction aphasia. In addition to word-finding problems, the hallmark of this form of aphasia is difficulty with spoken word repetition. It is associated with pathology concentrated in the left (dominant) hemisphere temporo-parietal junction (Rhorer et al., 2010), and is an example of a conduction disorder as it disconnects the speech comprehension areas from the speech production areas.

Diagnosis of PPA usually follows a two-stage process, outlined by Gorno-Tempini, Hillis, and Grossman (2011), with initial consideration given to whether the criteria for PPA are met, followed by evaluation of which subtype of PPA this may represent. Onset must be insidious and not better explained by another pathology (e.g. tumour, stroke), and aphasia must be the initial and most prominent presenting feature. Caution must be retained not to opt for identifying a subtype first, as language difficulties can present as part of typical DAT. For a diagnosis of PPA other common features of DAR need to be absent, the main exclusion criteria being (1) prominent episodic memory deficits, (2) non-verbal memory loss, and (3) visuospatial difficulties. If there is supporting evidence of atrophy, the diagnosis is referred to as imaging-supported, with a definite diagnosis only made with evidence of pathology which may become more feasible with the introduction of biomarkers. Identification of lvPPA is considered more problematic than for the other two forms, as the presentation is less distinct and is more likely to show some effects on other non-linguistic aspects of cognitive function (Marshall et al., 2018). There is some evidence emerging that it may be possible to distinguish DAT lvPPA from non-DAT lvPPA on the basis of linguistic presentation, but currently available tests are not able to do this clinically (Da Cuhna et al., 2022).

Frontal Variant DAT

Frontal variant DAT (FvDAT) is relatively rare, although difficulty with diagnosis may mean it is more common than is realised. In terms of the clinical presentation, it is difficult to distinguish from behavioural variant frontal temporal dementia (fvFTD), and may also get confused with VD (Sawyer et al., 2017). So far, the author has yet to identify a reliable means of diagnosing fvDAT clinically, although this may change with the increasing availability of biomarkers.

Limbic-Predominant Age-Related TDP-43 Encephalopathy

Limbic-Predominant Age-Related TDP-43 Encephalopathy (LATE) is not a form of DAT, but presents clinically in a manner very similar to DAT (Pao et al., 2011). Rather than the types of amyloid and tau proteins seen in DAT, LATE is associated with an abnormal variant of a tau protein called TDP-43 (Dickson et al., 1994), which is also implicated in FTD and motor neurone disease (McKenzie et al., 2007). The pathology associated with LATE is referred to as LATE-NC (Nelson et al., 2019) and is seen mainly in the brains of adults over the age of 80, with reports from post-mortem studies of occurrence in up to 50% of the brains of people in that age group (Nelson et al., 2019). As with DAT, LATE pathology can co-occur with other forms of pathology, such as Lewy bodies, Alzheimer-related pathology, and vascular pathology (Besser, Taylan, & Nelson, 2020). LATE often presents with unilateral hippocampal sclerosis, even when the distribution of LATE-NC is bilateral (Nelson et al., 2011). While LATE is undoubtedly an exciting topic for research, it can currently only be diagnosed post mortem. Although Nelson et al. (2019) suggest that there are differences in the cognitive profile of LATE when compared directly to people with DAT, it is uncertain whether LATE has a sufficiently distinct cognitive profile to distinguish it clinically from DAT.

Key Points

- Alzheimer's disease is the most common form of dementia, accounting for roughly 70% of cases.
- The prevalence increases with age, and many studies have reported a greater prevalence in women.
- Whilst there are some cases with a strong hereditary component, these are usually early-onset and the majority of late-onset cases are considered to be sporadic.
- Two abnormal proteins are associated with DAT: beta amyloid and tau. Which one is primary and whether one causes the other is uncertain. Other forms of dementia also feature abnormal variants of tau protein, but only DAT features both tau and beta amyloid.
- The primary deficit in Alzheimer's disease is the ability to create new memories (anterograde amnesia), with other functions being affected as the disease progresses.
- Tests of delayed memory are often most sensitive to DAT, followed by immediate memory. Long-term episodic memory (i.e. for events which occurred prior to the onset of the disorder) and semantic memory are often preserved in the early stages, but may be implicated as the disease progresses.
- There are a number of atypical variants of DAT, where the same abnormal proteins are present but have a different distribution throughout the cortex. Examples of these are PCA, logopenic PPA, and frontal variant DAT.
- LATE is a more recently identified proteinopathy which is not a form of DAT, but presents clinically in a very similar manner.

Appendix E Case Studies: DAT

Case Study: MM

MM was a 75-year-old male who presented to his GP with an 18-month history of forgetfulness, although his partner thought some indicators were present before this. Progression had been gradual. He gave examples of forgetting appointments and not recalling conversations after a few days. He recognised familiar people, although sometimes struggled with putting a name to a face. He was not particularly disturbed by this, although his wife was more concerned. He had some vascular risk factors, which were controlled with medications, and did not have any major lifestyle risk factors other than a fairly sedentary routine and a past history of smoking 20 cigarettes a day for 40 years. No irregularities were detected in his blood results, and a CT scan described 'involutional changes with no lobular predominance'. Basic activities of daily living were unimpaired, but he needed support with appointments and keeping track of his routines. IQcode rated by his wife suggested a change in function over the last ten years.

Neuropsychological assessment revealed mainly preserved cognitive abilities, but with a decline of more than two standard deviations in immediate and delayed memory. Also apparent in cognitive testing, his presentation at interview indicated some word-finding difficulties and circumlocutions. On the basis of a decline in function and a decline in cognition, a diagnosis of dementia was arrived at. Given the cognitive profile of a marked decline in immediate and delayed memory, probable DAT was the conclusion.

Case Study: DB

DB was an 82-year-old female with a progressive history of short-term memory problems which had developed gradually over a period of five years. She lived independently on her own, following the death of her husband five years earlier, at which point difficulties began to emerge. She was supported by her son and daughter, who lived nearby. Her daughter accompanied her to the appointment and provided background information.

DB described becoming less sociable, and having to make a concerted effort to see her friends even though she enjoyed their company. She had previously looked after the accounts for the local women's institute but now felt unable to keep track of these and had handed them over to another member. It subsequently became apparent that mistakes had been made for some time before she handed over responsibility.

DB had a relatively recent history of atrial fibrillation, and high blood pressure, both of which were now well controlled. She did not have any lifestyle risk factors. Her CT scan reported global atrophy, and mild-to-moderate small vessel disease, with evidence of a small, old area of infarction in the right frontal lobe.

Cognitive testing revealed evidence of a decline in delayed memory and executive function. There was also evidence of a decline in speed of information processing.

As there was evidence of change in instrumental activities of daily living (managing finances), and cognitive decline in more than one aspect of cognitive function, a diagnosis of dementia was given. Given the evidence of ischaemic change on her scan, a mixed presentation was considered most likely.

References

Aisen, P. S., Cummings, J., Jack, C. R., et al. (2017). On the path to 2025: Understanding the Alzheimer's disease continuum. *Alzheimer's Research & Therapy*, 9(1), 1–10.

Alzheimer, A. (1907). Über eine eigenaritage, schweren Erkrankung der Hirnrinde. *Allgemeine Zeitschrift für Psychiatrie und phychish-Gerichtliche Medizin (Berlin)*, 25, 1134.

Alzheimer Association (2022). Alzheimer's Disease Facts and Figures. Chicago, Illinois. Alzheimer Association, retrieved from Alzheimer's Disease Facts and Figures. www.alz.org/media/Documents/2022-Facts-and-Figures-Report_1.pdf.

Alzheimer's Society (2020). Can genes cause dementia? www.alzheimers.org.uk/about-dementia/risk-factors-and-prevention/alzheimers-disease-and-genes.

American Psychiatric Association (2013). *Diagnostic and Statistical Manual of Mental Disorders*, Fifth Edition, Text Revision. Washington, DC, American Psychiatric Association.

Arnaiz, E., & Almkvist, O. (2003). Neuropsychological features of mild cognitive impairment and preclinical Alzheimer's disease. *Acta Neurologica Scandinavica*, **107**, 4–41.

Bäckman, L., Jones, S., Berger, A. K., Laukka, E. J., & Small, B. J. (2005). Cognitive impairment in preclinical Alzheimer's disease: A meta-analysis. *Neuropsychology*, **19** (4), 520–31.

Bellenguez, C., Grenier-Boley, B., & Lambert, J. C. (2020). Genetics of Alzheimer's disease: Where we are, and where we are going. *Current Opinion in Neurobiology*, **61**, 40–8.

Bennett, D. A., Schneider, J. A., Arvanitakis, Z., et al. (2006). Neuropathology of older persons without cognitive impairment from two community-based studies. *Neurology*, **66** (12), 1837–44.

Besser, L. M., Teylan, M. A., & Nelson, P. T. (2020). Limbic predominant age-related TDP-43 encephalopathy (LATE): clinical and neuropathological associations. *Journal of Neuropathology & Experimental Neurology*, **79**(3), 305–13.

Bove, R., Secor, E., Chibnik, L. B., et al. (2014). Age at surgical menopause influences cognitive decline and Alzheimer pathology in older women. *Neurology*, **82**(3), 222–9.

Brenowitz, W. D., Hubbard, R. A., Keene, C. D., et al. (2017). Mixed neuropathologies and estimated rates of clinical progression in a large autopsy sample. *Alzheimer's & Dementia*, **13**(6), 654–62.

Braak, H., & Braak, E. (1996). Evolution of the neuropathology of Alzheimer's disease. *Acta Neurologica Scandinavica*, **94**(S165), 3–12.

Braak, H., Thal, D. R., Ghebremedhin, E., & Del Tredici, K. (2011). Stages of the pathologic process in Alzheimer disease: age categories from 1 to 100 years. *Journal of Neuropathology and Experimental Neurology*, **70**(11), 960–9.

Brion, J. P., Passareiro, H., Nunez, J., Flament-Durand, J. (1985). Mise en évidence immunologique de la protéine tau au niveau des lésions de dégénérescence neurofibrillaire de la maladie d'Alzheimer. *Arch Biol (Bruxelles)*, **95**, 229–35.

Cacace, R., Sleegers, K., & Van Broeckhoven, C. (2016). Molecular gee tics of early-onset Alzheimer's disease revisited. *Alzheimer's & Dementia*, **12**(6), 733–48.

Carlesimo, G. A., & Oscar-Berman, M. (1992). Memory deficits in Alzheimer's patients: A comprehensive review. *Neuropsychology Review*, **3**(2), 119–69.

Crutch, S. J., Schott, J. M., Rabinovici, G. D., et al. (2017). Consensus classification of posterior cortical atrophy. *Alzheimer's & Dementia: The Journal of the Alzheimer's Association*, **13**(8), 870–84.

Cummings, J. L., & Benson, D. F. (1992). *Dementia: A Clinical Approach*. Boston: Butterworth-Heineman.

Da Cunha, E., Plonka, A., Arslan, S., et al. (2022). Logogenic primary progressive aphasia or Alzheimer Disease: Contribution of acoustic markers in early differential diagnosis. *Life*, **12**(7), 933.

Delis, D. C., Kramer, J. H., Kaplan, E., & Ober, B. A. (2000). *California Verbal Learning Test-second edition: Adult version manual*. San Antonio: Psychological Corporation.

De Reuck, J., Maurage, C. A., Deramecourt, V., et al. (2018). Aging and cerebrovascular lesions in pure and in mixed neurodegenerative and vascular dementia brains: A neuropathological study. *Folia Neuropathologica*, **56**(2), 81–7.

Dickson, D. W., Davies, P., Bevona, C., et al. (1994). Hippocampal sclerosis: A common pathological feature of dementia in very old (4 or =80 years of age) humans. *Acta Neuropathologica*, **88**, 212–21.

Dubois, B., Villain, N., Frisoni, G. B., et al. (2021). Clinical diagnosis of Alzheimer's disease: recommendations of the International Working Group. *The Lancet Neurology*, **20**(6), 484–96.

Duchek, J. M., Cheney, M., Ferraro, F. R., & Storandt, M. (1991). Paired associate learning in senile dementia of the Alzheimer type. *Archives of neurology*, **48**(10),1038–40.

Enwefa, S., & Enwefa, R. (2018). Confrontation naming errors of Alzheimer's disease patients. *Online Journal of Neurology and Brain Disorders*, http://dx.doi.org/10.32474/OJNBD.2018.01.000117.

Fox, N. C., & Schott, J. M. (2004). Imaging cerebral atrophy: Normal ageing to Alzheimer's disease. *The Lancet*, **363**, 392–4.

Gao, S., Burney, H. N., Callahan, C. M., Purnell, C. E., & Hendrie, H. C. (2019). Incidence of dementia and Alzheimer disease over time: A meta-analysis. *Journal of the American Geriatrics Society*, **67**(7), 1361–9.

Glenner, G. G., Wong, C. W., Quaranta, V., & Eanes, E. D. (1984). The amyloid deposits in Alzheimer's disease: Their nature and pathogenesis. *Applied Pathology*, **2**(6), 357–69.

Gorno-Tempini, M. L., Dronkers, N. F., Rankin, K. P., et al. (2004). Cognition and anatomy in three variants of primary progressive aphasia. *Annals of Neurology: Official Journal of the American Neurological Association and the Child Neurology Society*, **55**(3), 335–46.

Gorno-Tempini, M. L., Hillis, A. E., Weintraub, S., et al. (2011). Classification of primary progressive aphasia and its variants. *Neurology*, **76**(11), 1006–14.

Gumus, M., Multani, N., Mack, M. L., Tartaglia, M. C., & Alzheimer's Disease Neuroimaging Initiative (2021). Progression of neuropsychiatric symptoms in young-onset versus late-onset Alzheimer's disease. *GeroScience*, **43**(1), 213–23.

Hardy, J. A., & Higgins, G. A. (1992). Alzheimer's disease: The amyloid cascade hypothesis. *Science*, **256**(5054), 184–5.

Henderson, V. W., & Sherwin, B. (2007). Surgical versus natural menopause. *Menopause*, **14**(3), 572–9.

Henry, J. D., Crawford, J. R., & Phillips, L. H. (2004). Verbal fluency performance in dementia of the Alzheimer's type: a meta-analysis. *Neuropsychologia*, **42**(9), 1212–22.

Herrup, K. (2015). The case for rejecting the amyloid cascade hypothesis. *Nature Neuroscience*, **18**(6), 794–9.

Hicks, E. B., Ahsan, N., Bhandari, A., et al. (2021). Associations of visual paired associative learning task with global cognition and its potential usefulness as a screening tool for Alzheimer's dementia. *International Psychogeriatrics*, **33**(11), 1135–44.

Hof, P. R., Vogt, B. A., Bouras, C., & Morrison, J. H. (1997). Atypical form of Alzheimer's disease with prominent posterior cortical atrophy: A review of lesion distribution and circuit disconnection in cortical visual pathways. *Vision Research*, **37**(24), 3609–25.

Jack, C. R., Jr, Bennett, D. A., Blennow, K., et al. (2018). NIA-AA Research Framework: Toward a biological definition of Alzheimer's disease. *Alzheimer's & Dementia : The Journal of the Alzheimer's Association*, **14**(4), 535–62.

Jack, C. R., Wiste, H. J., Weigand, S. D., et al. (2014). Age-specific population frequencies of cerebral β-amyloidosis and neurodegeneration among people with normal cognitive function aged 50–89 years: A cross-sectional study. *The Lancet Neurology*, **13**(10), 997–1005.

James, B. D., Bennett, D. A., Boyle, P. A., Leurgans, S., & Schneider, J. A. (2017). Dementia from Alzheimer disease and mixed pathologies in the oldest old. *Journal of the American Medical Association*, **307**(17), 1798–800.

Johnson, D. K., Storandt, M., Balota, D. A. (2003). Discourse analysis of logical memory recall in normal aging and in dementia of the Alzheimer type. *Neuropsychology*, **17**, 82–92.

Kapasi, A., DeCarli, C., & Schneider, J. A. (2017). Impact of multiple pathologies on the threshold for clinically overt dementia. *Acta Neuropathologica*, **134**(2), 171–86.

Koedam, E., Lauffer, V., van der Vlies, A., et al. (2010). Early-versus late-onset A;zheimer's disease: More than age alone. *Journal of Alzheimer's Disease*, **19**(4), 1401–8.

Lukatela, K., Malloy, P., Jenkins, M., & Cohen, R. (1998). The naming deficit in early

Alzheimer's and vascular dementia. *Neuropsychology*, **12**(4), 565–72.

Maccioni, R., Farias, G., Morales, I., & Navarette, L. (2010). The revitalized tau hypothesis on Alzheimer's disease. *Archives of Medical Research*, **41**(3), 226–31.

Mackenzie, I. R., Bigio, E. H., Ince, P. G., et al. (2007). Pathological TDP-43 distinguishes sporadic amyotrophic lateral sclerosis from amyotrophic lateral sclerosis with SOD1 mutations. *Annals of Neurology:Official Journal of the American Neurological Association and the Child Neurology Society*, **61**(5), 427–34.

McMonagle, P., Deering, F., Berliner, Y., & Kertesz, A. (2006). The cognitive profile of posterior cortical atrophy. *Neurology*, **66**(3), 331–8.

Marshall, C. R., Hardy, C. J., Volkmer, A., et al. (2018). Primary progressive aphasia: A clinical approach. *Journal of Neurology*, **265**(6), 1474–90.

McKhann, G., Drachman, D., Folstein, M., et al. (1984). Clinical diagnosis of Alzheimer's disease: Report of the NINCDS-ADRDA Work Group under the auspices of Department of Health and Human Services Task Force on Alzheimer's Disease. *Neurology*, **34**, 939–44.

McKhann, G. M., Knopman, D. S., Chertkow, H., et al. (2011). The diagnosis of dementia due to Alzheimer's disease: Recommendations from the National Institute on Aging-Alzheimer's Association workgroups on diagnostic guidelines for Alzheimer's disease. *Alzheimer's & Dementia*, **7**(3), 263–9.

Mendez, M. F., Ghajarania, M., & Perryman, K. M. (2002). Posterior cortical atrophy: Clinical characteristics and differences compared to Alzheimer's disease. *Dementia and Geriatric Cognitive Disorders*, **14**(1), 33–40.

Mesulam, M. M., Wieneke, C., Thompson, C., Rogalski, E., & Weintraub, S. (2012). Quantitative classification of primary progressive aphasia at early and mild impairment stages. *Brain*, **135**(5), 1537–53.

Nelson, P. T., Dickson, D. W., Trojanowski, J. Q., et al. (2019). Limbic-predominant age-related TDP-43 encephalopathy (LATE): Consensus working group report. *Brain*, **142**(6), 1503–27.

Nelson, P. T., Head, E., Schmitt, F. A., et al. (2011). Alzheimer's disease is not 'brain aging': neuropathological, genetic, and epidemiological human studies. *Acta Neuropathologica*, **121**(5), 571–587.

Nelson, P. T., Schmitt, F. A., Lin, Y., et al. (2011). Hippocampal sclerosis in advanced age: Clinical and pathological features. *Brain*, **134** (5), 1506–18.

Niu, H., Álvarez-Álvarez, I., Guillén-Grima, F., & Aguinaga-Ontoso, I. (2017). Prevalence and incidence of Alzheimer's disease in Europe: A meta-analysis. *Neurología*, **32**(8), 523–32.

Pache, M., Smeets, C. H., Gasio, P. F., et al. (2003). Colour vision deficiencies in Alzheimer's disease. *Age and Ageing*, **32**(4), 422–6.

Pao, W. C., Dickson, D. W., Crook, J. E., et al. (2011). Hippocampal sclerosis in the elderly: Genetic and pathologic findings, some mimicking Alzheimer disease clinically. *Alzheimer Disease and Associated Disorders*, **25**, 364–8.

Price, J. L., & Morris, J. C. (1999). Tangles and plaques in nondemented aging and 'preclinical' Alzheimer's disease. *Annals of Neurology: Official Journal of the American Neurological Association and The Child Neurology Society*, **45**(3), 358–68.

Rabin, L. A., Paré, N., Saykin, A. J., et al. (2009). Differential memory test sensitivity for diagnosing amnestic mild cognitive impairment and predicting conversion to Alzheimer's disease. *Aging, Neuropsychology, and Cognition*, **16**(3), 357–76.

Rajan, K. B., Weuve, J., Barnes, L. L., Wilson, R. S., & Evans, D. A. (2019). Prevalence and incidence of clinically diagnosed Alzheimer's disease dementia from 1994 to 2012 in a population study. *Alzheimer's & Dementia: The Journal of the Alzheimer's Association*, **15**(1), 1–7.

Rajan, K. B., Weuve, J., Barnes, L. L., et al. (2021). Population estimate of people with clinical Alzheimer's disease and mild cognitive impairment in the United States

(2020–2060). *Alzheimer's & Dementia: The Journal of the Alzheimer's Association*, **17** (12), 1966–75.

Rohrer, J. D., Ridgway, G. R., Crutch, S. J., et al. (2010). Progressive logopenic/phonological aphasia: erosion of the language network. *Neuroimage*, **49**(1), 984–93.

Rossor, M. N., Fox, N. C., Mummery, C. J., Schott, J. M., & Warren, J. D. (2010). The diagnosis of young-onset dementia. *The Lancet. Neurology*, **9**(8), 793–806.

Saunders, A. M., Blennow, K., Breteler, M. M. B. et al. (1993). Association of apolipoprotein E allele ε4 with late-onset familial and sporadic Alzheimer's disease. *Neurology*, **43**(8), 1467.

Sawyer, R. P., Rodriguez-Porcel, F., Hagen, M., Shatz, R., & Espay, A. J. (2017). Diagnosing the frontal variant of Alzheimer's disease: A clinician's yellow brick road. *Journal of Clinical Movement Disorders*, **4**, 2.

Schmidt, M. (1996). *Rey Auditory and Verbal Learning Test: A handbook*. Los Angeles: Western Psychological Services.

Schöll, M., Lockhart, S. N., Schonhaut, D. R., et al. (2016). PET imaging of tau deposition in the aging human brain. *Neuron*, **89**(5), 971–82.

Schott, J. M., & Crutch, S. J. (2019). Posterior cortical atrophy. *Continuum*, **25**(1), 52–75.

Silbert, L. C., Quinn, J. F., Moore, M. M., et al. (2003). Changes in premorbid brain volume predict Alzheimer's disease pathology. *Neurology*, **61**(4), 487–92.

Spina, S., La Joie, R., Petersen, C., et al. (2021). Comorbid neuropathological diagnoses in early versus late-onset Alzheimer's disease. *Brain: A Journal of Neurology*, **144**(7), 2186–98.

Stanley, K., & Walker, Z. (2014). Do patients with young onset Alzheimer's disease deteriorate faster than those with late onset Alzheimer's disease? A review of the literature. *International Psychogeriatrics*, **26** (12), 1945–53.

Stroop, J. R. (1935). Studies of interference in serial verbal reaction. *Journal of Experimental Psychology*, **18**, 643–62.

Stute, P., Wienges, J., Koller, A. S., et al. (2021). Cognitive health after menopause: Does menopausal hormone therapy affect it? *Best Practice & Research Clinical Endocrinology & Metabolism*, **35**(6), 101565.

Tang, M. X., Jacobs, D., Stern, Y., et al. (1996). Effect of oestrogen during menopause on risk and age at onset of Alzheimer's disease. *The Lancet*, **348**(9025), 429–32.

Tang-Wai, D. F., Josephs, K. A., Boeve, B. F., et al. (2003). Pathologically confirmed corticobasal degeneration presenting with visuospatial dysfunction. *Neurology*, **61**, 1134–5.

Tom, S. E., Hubbard, R. A., Crane, P. K., et al. (2015). Characterization of dementia and Alzheimer's disease in an older population: Updated incidence and life expectancy with and without dementia. *American Journal of Public Health*, **105**(2), 408–13.

Tremont, D., Halpert, S., Javorsky, D. J., & Stern, R. A. (2000). Differential impact of executive dysfunction on verbal list learning and story recall. *The Clinical Neuropsychologist*, **14**, 295–302.

van der Flier, W. M., Pijnenburg, Y. A., Fox, N. C., & Scheltens, P. (2011). Early-onset versus late-onset Alzheimer's disease: The case of the missing APOE ε4 allele. *The Lancet Neurology*, **10**(3), 280–8.

Vellas, B., Carrillo, M. C., Sampaio, C., et al. (2013). Designing drug trials for Alzheimer's disease: What we have learned from the release of the phase III antibody trials: A report from the EU/US/CTAD Task Force. *Alzheimers & Dementia*, **9**(4), 438–444.

Wu, M., Li, M., Yuan, J., et al. (2020). Postmenopausal hormone therapy and Alzheimer's disease, dementia, and Parkinson's disease: A systematic review and time-response meta-analysis. *Pharmacological Research*, **155**, p.104693.

Zakzanis, K. K., Leach, L., & Kaplan, E. (1999). *Neuropsychological Differential Diagnosis*. Lisse: Swets & Zeitlinger.

Vascular Dementia

Vascular cognitive impairment (VCI) occurs as a result of problems with blood supply to the brain, and encompasses stroke, vascular MCI, and vascular dementia (VaD) (Dichgans & Leys, 2017). VaD is considered to be the second most common cause of dementia after Alzheimer's disease (DAT), accounting for approximately 20% of cases (Gorelick et al., 2011). Vascular pathology frequently co-occurs with Alzheimer pathology, in which case it is referred to as 'mixed dementia', and it has been suggested that the combination of DAT and VaD is the single biggest cause of later life dementia (Smith, 2017). VCI, or VaD, is not a single entity, as there are a number of different cerebrovascular disorders which can lead to cognitive decline and, ultimately, dementia. There have been various proposals for how to categorise the different forms of VCI/VaD. The Vascular Impairment of Cognition Classification Consensus Study (Skrobot et al., 2018) recommends the following four subtypes of VaD:

1. Post-stroke dementia
2. Subcortical ischaemic VaD
3. Multi-infarct (cortical) dementia
4. Mixed dementia (e.g. VaD with AD)

It is of course possible for someone to fall into more than one of these categories, for example by having ischaemic changes in both the cortex and subcortical areas.

Prevalence and Incidence

The prevalence of VaD increases with age and varies between countries, from 1.2 to 4.2% of the population over 65, with an incidence of 6–12 cases per 1,000 persons per year (Herbert & Brayne, 1995). There is an exponential age-related rise in the rates of VaD, with the risk doubling every five years from the age of 65 (Jorm & Jolley, 1998). Unlike DAT, where higher rates are reported for women, gender differences are not reliably found for rates of VaD (Andersen et al., 1999), although a greater age-adjusted incidence rate in men has been reported (Yoshitake et al., 1995).

Incidence of VaD is greatly increased following a stroke, with roughly 15–30% of stroke patients developing dementia within a few months, and a further 20–25% over a longer time period (Pendlebury & Rothwell, 2009). Mean survival time is 3–5 years, with cardiovascular and cerebrovascular factors being the main cause of death (Kua et al., 2014). There is a degree of variation between countries, as VaD accounts for 50% of all dementias in China and Japan (Román et al., 2004), whereas in Europe and North America DAT is more common.

Whilst progression is common, it should be noted that some people remain stable following a vascular event, and there can also be a period of improvement (Rasquin, Lodder, & Verhey, 2005).

The conventional wisdom is that, unlike other forms of dementia, VaD follows a stepwise and fluctuating pattern of onset, with periods of stability or even improvement (Hachinski & Bowler, 1993). Whilst this may accurately describe the pattern seen with multi-infarct dementia, it may not represent other forms of cerebrovascular disorder such as small vessel disease (SVD), which is associated with a more gradual onset (Sachdev et al., 2014).

It should be noted that VaD most commonly co-occurs with other pathologies such as DAT, and 'pure' VaD is now considered to be relatively rare (Hulette et al., 1997).

Pathology

VCI and VaD are forms of cerebrovascular disease, which refers to problems with blood supply to the brain. As with stroke, the way this occurs is via (1) blood vessels becoming blocked (ischaemia), and/or from (2) bleeding (haemorrhage). Following one or both of these events, areas of the brain do not get sufficient blood supply, which results in cell death. There are, however, a number of different ways that this comes about, and a number of different possible presentations of VaD, with the site and size of lesions being important for the clinical consequences. Multi-infarct dementia, which arises from a series of small and larger strokes, was initially considered to be the main cause of VaD (Hachinski, Lassen, & Marshall, 1974). However, it is now recognised that VaD can arise from a number of different sources, including strategic single infarcts, non-infarction white matter lesions, haemorrhages, and hypoperfusion (Sachdev et al., 2014). The most common cause of VaD is currently considered to be SVD, which progresses via an accumulation of white matter lesions and lacunes (fluid-filled spaces) (Dichgens & Leys, 2017). These can often be identified via imaging, particularly MRI scans, but are a relatively common finding from middle age onwards. They are found in approximately 50% of people aged 45 (Wen et al., 2009) and 95% of people aged 80 or over (de Leeuw et al., 2001). The question therefore arises of what level of white matter lesions should be considered clinically significant. Unfortunately, there is as yet no consensus on this, and the various diagnostic criteria have different requirements. Price et al. (2005) recommended that at least 25% of the white matter should be affected for a diagnosis of VaD, whereas Sachdev et al. (2014) prefer a less strict guideline that white matter lesions should be 'extensive and confluent'.

Strategic infarcts refer to a single or limited number of lesions to key areas which can result in widespread cognitive impairment. This includes structures such as the thalamus, angular gyrus, and basal ganglia (Dichgans & Leys, 2017).

Alongside the age-related risk of accumulating vascular lesions, other forms of neuropathology are often found in the brains of older adults. In the general population without dementia, the prevalence of cortical infarcts, lacunar infarcts, microbleeds, and beta amyloid protein all increase with age, so it is likely that most older patients presenting with cognitive decline will have multiple contributing factors (Wolters & Ikram, 2019).

VCI and Alzheimer's Disease (Mixed Dementia)

There is an increasing recognition that a mixture of AD and vascular pathology may be the norm in most cases of late-onset dementia (i.e. in persons over 80 years of age). Although vascular lesions can co-occur with any form of degenerative dementia, they are more commonly found with AD than any other form of pathology (Toledo et al., 2013). The two forms of pathology are considered to have a synergistic effect (Zerky et al., 2002), resulting in a greater level of cognitive impairment than would be expected from each pathology in isolation. One of the first illustrations of this came from the 'nun' study (Snowden, 2001), which is an ongoing research project following up an order of nuns as they age and examining their brains post-mortem. In the initial studies, some nuns showed little evidence of cognitive decline whilst alive, but were found to have quite advanced AD post-mortem, whereas others developed more severe cognitive decline with relatively little Alzheimer pathology. Those who developed greater cognitive decline and dementia had a higher level of vascular lesions, particularly in the basal ganglia, thalamus, and white matter (Snowden et al., 1997).

Although there is no direct evidence for a cause-and-effect relationship between the two types of pathology, mechanisms whereby this could take place have been proposed (Fierini, 2020; Klohs, 2019; Niwa et al., 2002). It is known that vascular risk factors are also associated with AD, and there are mechanisms whereby AD can cause vascular lesions, such as cerebral amyloid angiopathy, where amyloid protein deposits build up in cerebral blood vessels, although this condition is also common in the general older adult population (Biffi & Greenberg, 2011). There are also cases where vascular changes precede the development of DAT, which have led to the suggestion that it has a causal role (Attems & Jellinger, 2014; Klohs, 2019). Another theory is that inflammation may be a common factor, with both vascular lesions and proteinopathies giving rise to and arising from inflammation (Encui & Popescu, 2013). It should, however, be noted that treatment with anti-inflammatory medication has yet to be demonstrated as an effective treatment for halting/slowing cognitive decline (Jordan et al., 2020).

Consensus on clinical diagnosis of mixed dementia, or even how to best describe it, is lacking at the moment. DSM-V covers this briefly under the heading of Mild or Major Neurocognitive Disorder due to Multiple Etiologies. Their criteria consist of (1) meeting the criteria for mild or major neurocognitive disorder, (2) evidence from history, physical examination, and laboratory tests of multiple aetiologies, and (3) cognitive deficits are not better explained by another mental disorder, or occur within the context of a delirium. The VASCOG diagnostic criteria (Sachdev et al., 2014) recommend the clinician make a diagnosis of mild or major neurocognitive disorder and then decide which is the most prominent pathology.

The Hachinski Ischemic Scale (Hachinski et al., 1975) is a 13-item scale, on which each item is assigned a score. It was designed to diagnose VaD, with a reported sensitivity of 89% and specificity of 89% (Knopman et al., 2001). It has been found to reliably distinguish between pure AD and VaD, and between AD and mixed dementia: it does not distinguish between mixed dementia and VaD (Moroney et al., 1997). Although questions have been raised regarding the validity of the scale, particularly in relation to mixed dementia (Gräsel, Cameron, & Lehrl, 1990) and it was designed with the intention of identifying multi-infarct dementia rather than SVD, it is still widely used. The 13-item version can be found in Appendix G at the end of this chapter.

Risk Factors

Although there is no direct treatment for VaD, it is potentially one of the more preventable forms as it shares risk factors with stroke and heart disease, some of which are modifiable. As mentioned earlier, stroke is a major risk factor for developing VaD. Transient ischaemic attacks (TIA) with an effect on cognition are associated with a 5-fold increased risk of developing dementia within 5 years (Pendlebury et al., 2011). Vascular risk factors include hypertension, ischaemic heart disease, atrial fibrillation, raised cholesterol, diabetes, and obesity (Gorelick et al., 2011). Lifestyle risk factors include alcohol intake, diet, obesity, and smoking, whereas engaging in education, physical activity, and complex mental activity can be protective (Sachdev et al., 2014).

Although risk factors increase the likelihood of developing VCI, they are not diagnostic as they also increase the risk of developing other forms of dementia such as AD (Purnell et al., 2009). The presence of risk factors does not necessarily mean the person will develop VCI, and the possibility of reducing rates of dementia by addressing modifiable risk factors will be discussed in Chapter 12.

Genetics

There is a well-known, albeit rare, genetic subtype of VCI called cerebral autosomal dominant arteriopathy with subcortical infarcts and leukoencephalopathy (CADASIL). This is a gradually progressing form of SVD, with symptoms typically developing between the ages of 30 and 40, characterised by cognitive decline and recurrent strokes (Alzheimer Society, 2022). It is associated with the NOTCH3 gene, which is autosomal dominant (Ferrante, Cudrici, & Boehm, 2019), meaning it can be inherited from one parent and can be passed on equally to males and females. Genetic testing would be advised for anybody presenting with possible CADASIL.

Although there have not been many studies on genetics and VCI, some genes have been identified as having an association, although the associations are not strong and not exclusive to VCI. For instance, APOE e4 has an association with VCI, but is also closely associated with DAT and cardiovascular disease (O'Brien & Thomas, 2015).

Cognitive Profile

Given the number of different possible causes, there is not a generic cognitive profile for VCI. Someone with post-stroke dementia is likely to have a different profile to someone with SVD, which in turn is likely to differ from someone with a single strategic infarct. However, studies have been carried out using neuropsychological assessments which indicate some common features which could help distinguish SVD from DAT. SVD is associated with a subcortical profile, with the greatest deficits being seen in speed of information processing and executive function (Vasquez & Zakzanis, 2015). Sachdev et al. (2004) compared patients with VCI to those with VaD, finding that VaD patients showed more severe impairment but retained the same overall pattern of strengths and weaknesses. It is likely that this pattern of impairment arises from impoverished connections between the basal ganglia, thalamus, and frontal lobes.

When compared to patients with DAT, patients with SVD typically show a less severe memory deficit (Graham, Emery, & Hodges, 2004; Traykov et al., 2005). Preserved recognition memory has also been reported as feature of SVD, which is not seen in DAT (e.g. Tierney et al., 2001). Patients with SVD can also benefit more from the use of cues, which is consistent with the idea that the memory impairment in VCI is related to retrieval, whereas in DAT it is a deficit in encoding (Cerciello et al., 2017).

Herbert et al. (2014) compared verbal fluency performance between patients with SVD, DAT, and healthy controls. SVD patients were equally impaired at both letter and semantic fluency when compared to controls, whereas DAT patients showed a deficit in semantic fluency only. On the basis of performance on this test, they were able to correctly classify 80% of SVD patients and 92% of DAT patients.

Whilst these patterns of impairment may be typical of patients presenting with SVD, it should be borne in mind that the presence of multiple infarcts would be likely to produce some focal deficits – for example, aphasia following a left middle cerebral artery infarct, sensory inattention following a right middle cerebral artery infarct, and memory problems following a posterior cortical artery infarct.

Neuropsychiatric Signs

Depression is common amongst older adults and has been reported to occur in 31% of patients in the first five years following a stroke (Ayerbe et al., 2013). Late-onset depression is frequently associated with ischaemic changes, which are not seen in early-onset depression (Krishnan, 2002). This relationship between vascular lesions and late-onset depression led to the concept of vascular depression (Alexopoulos et al., 1999). It is usually treatment resistant, and is also associated with a decline in executive function, presumably arising from damage to cortico-striatal pathways.

Although DSM-V does not have a diagnostic category for vascular depression, the phrase is used when describing features which support a diagnosis of VaD (American Psychiatric Association, 2013, p. 622). It is therefore unsurprising that depression is common in VCI and VCD. Tiel et al. (2015) carried out a systematic review of neuropsychiatric symptoms in VaD, and reported that depression and apathy were equally common amongst patients with subcortical SVD and those with cortical lesions as well. These were less common in VCI patients without dementia.

Anxiety is also common in VaD, and seemingly more common than in DAT (Ballard et al., 2000). A history of anxiety is also a risk factor for the development of both VaD and DAT (Becker et al., 2018).

Imaging

Given the emphasis on establishing evidence of cerebrovascular disease, imaging plays an important role in the diagnosis of VCI and VaD. CT scans are widely available, and are able to identify atrophy, established infarcts and extensive white matter lesions, but MRI is preferred as it allows for better identification of the degree, extent, and location of vascular lesions (O'Brien & Thomas, 2015). MRI is better at detecting SVD, the hallmarks of which are white matter hypointensities (WMH) and lacunar infarcts. Although enlarged periventricular spaces and brain atrophy are also hallmarks of SVD, these are also seen in degenerative disorders (Iadecola et al., 2019).

New developments in imaging technology will be covered in Chapter 13.

Diagnostic Criteria

There have been several different diagnostic criteria for VaD, and now for VCI. There are some significant differences between them in terms of emphasis, to the extent that they may not be diagnosing the same thing, although they all share three core elements:

1. Evidence of cognitive decline
2. Evidence of cerebrovascular disease

3. Evidence of a causal relationship (i.e. the extent and location of the vascular burden should be commensurate with the level of cognitive decline)

The National Institute of Neurological Disorders and Stroke-Association Internationale pour la Recherché et l'Enseignement en Neurosciences (NINDS-AIREN) (Román et al., 1993) criteria have been highly influential, but were written from the perspective of multi-infarct dementia being the most likely cause of VCI and also required a memory deficit to be present. The criteria outlined here are based on the International Society for Vascular Behavioural and Cognitive Disorders (VASCOG) guidelines (Sachdev et al., 2014), which are intended to align with DSM-V (American Psychiatric Association, 2013). The VASCOG guidelines recommend following DSM-V for identifying the presence of major neurocognitive disorder (dementia) or mild neurocognitive disorder (MCI) (covered in Chapter 2). Evidence for cognitive decline requires both a subjective report (patient or informant), as well as an objective decline established through formal testing.

Evidence to support a predominantly vascular aetiology are listed as follows.

1. Clinical features:

In the context of a stepwise/fluctuating pattern of onset

- Documented history of a stroke, with cognitive decline temporally associated with the event
- Physical signs consistent with stroke (e.g. hemiparesis, lower facial weakness, sensory deficit including visual field defect)

In the context of gradual onset with a slow course in the absence of a history of stroke or TIA, a decline should be apparent in speed of information processing, complex attention, and executive function. In addition to this, evidence is required for one of the following:

- Early presence of gait disturbance
- Increased urinary urgency or other urinary symptoms not caused by urologic disease
- Personality and mood changes

2. Evidence from neuroimaging, which should take the form of *one* of the following:

- One large vessel infarct for MCI, two or more for VaD
- Extensive or strategically placed infarct, usually in the thalamus or basal ganglia
- Two or more lacunar infarcts outside the brainstem, or 1–2 lacunes which are either strategically placed or combined with extensive white matter lesions
- Extensive and confluent white matter lesions
- Strategically placed intracerebral haemorrhage, or two or more intracerebral haemorrhages
- A combination of the above

Exclusion criteria apply to both vascular MCI and VaD.

- History of early memory or other focal cognitive deficits in the absence of focal lesions on scan or history of vascular events. Parkinsonian features suggestive of dementia with Lewy bodies. History suggestive of other neurological disease which could affect cognition, such as multiple sclerosis
- CT or MRI scan shows absent or minimal vascular lesions
- Other medical disorders which could account for cognitive problems (e.g. brain tumour, encephalitis). Major depression temporally linked with the onset of cognitive problems. Evidence of toxins or metabolic abnormalities

When both clinical and imaging criteria are met, a diagnosis of probable VCI/VaD can be made. In the relatively rare instances of a genetic variant such as CADASIL, clinical and genetic criteria should be met. When clinical criteria are met, but imaging was not available, the diagnosis may be possible VCI/VaD. However, if imaging was available but did not support a vascular underpinning, VCI/VaD cannot be diagnosed.

Key Points

- VCI is an umbrella term for disorders of the blood supply to the brain which result in cognitive decline. VaD is the most severe form.
- VaD is considered to be the second most common cause of dementia after Alzheimer's disease, and the risk of developing it increases with age.
- A range of disorders can lead to VCI, with differing presentations. Initially, multi-infarct dementia was considered to be the most common subtype, which is characterised by a stepwise, fluctuating progression. However, it is now thought that SVD is the most common subtype, which is characterised by a gradual, steady progression.
- Alzheimer's disease and cerebrovascular disease commonly co-occur. The overall effect of cognitive function is likely to reflect a combination of these two pathologies. It has also been proposed that the presence of one of these forms of pathology had a causative effect on the development of the other.
- Risk factors for VCI (and Alzheimer's disease) are the same as for stroke and heart disease, some of which are modifiable. This means it is potentially preventable in some cases.
- Although there is not one cognitive profile for all forms, there is a profile associated with SVD. This consists of primary deficits in executive function, speed of processing, and attention, with a relative preservation of memory. Letter and category fluency are equally impaired, whereas category fluency is often more affected in Alzheimer's disease.
- Depression and anxiety are relatively common.
- MRI scans are the preferred option for identifying hallmarks of vascular change.
- Numerous diagnostic criteria have been proposed, which do not entirely overlap. However, the common theme is (1) evidence of cognitive decline, (2) evidence of cerebrovascular disease. The extent of the cerebrovascular disease should be considered sufficient to account for the cognitive changes.
- If imaging evidence is not available, a diagnosis of possible VaD can be given. However, if there is imaging data which does not support the presence of vascular change, this diagnosis cannot be given.

Appendix F Case Studies

Case Study: Mrs G

Mrs G was an 82-year-old female, who presented to her GP, at the request of her daughter, with a complaint of gradually progressing memory problems. This was initially put down to age-related absent-mindedness. She lived with and was the main carer for her husband, who had been diagnosed with Alzheimer's disease two years previously. Mrs G always kept track of her husband's medical appointments, but over the last year there were a number of examples of missed appointments or attending on the wrong day. She had previously kept track of their finances via online banking, but now required assistance from her daughter to do this. She also showed some confusion with names of familiar people. Mrs G was generally healthy, although she had experienced some cardiac problems and high blood pressure, both of which were well controlled with medication. Although Mrs G reported low mood, this was attributed to the stress of being a carer for her husband.

Mrs G agreed to attend a neuropsychology assessment. Her cognitive profile showed a primary deficit in delayed memory and executive function, the tests for both of which were greater than 2 standard deviations lower than expected on the basis of estimated premorbid ability. An MRI scan revealed evidence of generalised atrophy, although it was not specified whether this was within age-related limits. There was also evidence of medial temporal lobe atrophy. There was also evidence of an old infarct in her left parietal lobe, and diffuse white matter lesions consistent with SVD.

Despite the identified hallmarks of vascular changes, Mrs G's neuropsychological and clinical profiles were more consistent with Alzheimer's disease. Consequently, a diagnosis of mixed dementia was arrived at.

Case Study: Mr F

Mr F was a 69-year-old man with a number of physical health problems, including atrial fibrillation, high blood pressure, and elevated cholesterol. His wife had noticed some decline in function, in that he got muddled in relation to financial matters and struggled to work the mobile phone bought for him by his daughter. Mr F had smoked 20 cigarettes a day for many years, and had only stopped five years ago following a bout of pneumonia. He had also been a steady drinker throughout his life, drinking two bottles of whisky a week, and occasionally a third bottle over the weekend. His current alcohol consumption had reduced greatly, and he now rarely exceeded 14 units a week. He was overweight and lived a sedentary lifestyle.

Mr F's wife felt there had been a steady deterioration over the last five years, mainly noticeable as an inability to organise his diary and plan for upcoming appointments and events. He did not report difficulty following conversations nor being able to follow the plot of films. Neuropsychological assessment demonstrated reduced speed of information processing (> 2 standard deviations) and executive function (2 standard deviations). Immediate and delayed memory were 1–1.5 standard deviations lower than expected.

Mr F's MRI scan showed the presence of diffuse white matter lesions, consistent with 'moderate small vessel disease'. There was some global atrophy, but not lobar predominance.

Mr F was given a diagnosis of VaD as his day-to-day function had declined and his neuropsychological assessment indicated a decline of more than two standard deviations in two aspects of cognition, neither of which was memory. There was evidence of ischaemic changes on his MRI scan, but no evidence of medial temporal lobe atrophy. The absence of evidence for an Alzheimer-type component led to VaD being considered more likely than a mixed dementia.

Appendix G The Hachinski Ischaemic Scale

Abrupt onset of symptoms	2
Stepwise deterioration (e.g. decline-stability-decline)	1
Fluctuating course	2
Nocturnal confusion	1
Personality relatively preserved	1
Depression	1
Somatic complaints (e.g. body aches, chest pain)	1
Emotional lability	1
History or presence of hypertension	1
History of stroke	2
Evidence of coexisting atherosclerosis (e.g. peripheral artery disease, myocardial infarction)	1
Focal neurologic symptoms (e.g. hemiparesis, homonymous hemianopia, aphasia)	2
Focal neurologic signs (e.g. unilateral weakness, sensory loss, asymmetric reflexes, Babinski sign)	2

A total score of less than or equal to 4 indicates Alzheimer's disease, and a score of greater than or equal to 7 indicates multi-infarct dementia. A score of 5 or 6 is labelled as indeterminate, and is sometimes interpreted as mixed dementia.

References

Alexopoulos, G. S., Bruce, M. L., Silbersweig, D., Kalayam, B., & Stern, E. (2022). Vascular depression: A new view of late-onset depression. *Dialogues in Clinical Neuroscience*, **1**(2), 68–80.

Alzheimer's Society (2022). CADASIL is a rare, inherited type of vascular disease that can cause dementia. www.alzheimers.org.uk/about-dementia/types-dementia/cadasil.

American Psychiatric Association. *Diagnostic and Statistical Manual of Mental Disorders*. 5th edition. (2013). Washington, DC: American Psychiatric Publishing.

Andersen, K., Launer, L. J., Dewey, M. E., et al. (1999). Gender differences in the incidence of AD and vascular dementia: The EURODEM Studies. *Neurology*, **53**(9), 1992.

Attems, J., & Jellinger, K. A. (2014). The overlap between vascular disease and Alzheimer's disease-lessons from pathology. *BMC Medicine*, **12**(1), 1–12.

Ayerbe, L., Ayis, S., Wolfe, C. D., & Rudd, A. G. (2013). Natural history, predictors and outcomes of depression after stroke: Systematic review and meta-analysis. *The British Journal of Psychiatry*, **202**(1), 14–21.

Ballard, C., Neill, D., O'Brien, J., et al. (2000). Anxiety, depression and psychosis in vascular dementia: Prevalence and associations. *Journal of Affective Disorders*, **59**(2), 97–106.

Biffi, A., & Greenberg, S. M. (2011). Cerebral amyloid angiopathy: A systematic review. *Journal of Clinical Neurology*, **7**(1), 1–9.

Cerciello, M., Isella, V., Proserpi, A., & Papagno, C. (2017). Assessment of free and cued recall in Alzheimer's disease and vascular and frontotemporal dementia with 24-item Grober and Buschke test. *Neurological Sciences*, **38**(1), 115–22.

De Leeuw, F. E., de Groot, J. C., Achten, E., et al. (2001). Prevalence of cerebral white matter lesions in elderly people: A population based magnetic resonance imaging study. The Rotterdam Scan Study. *Journal of Neurology, Neurosurgery & Psychiatry*, **70**(1), 9–14.

Dichgans, M., & Leys, D. (2017). Vascular cognitive impairment. *Circulation Research*, **120**(3), 573–91.

Enciu, A. M., & Popescu, B. O. (2013). Is there a causal link between inflammation and dementia? *BioMedical Research International*, Article ID 316495. http://dx.doi.org/10.1155/2013/316495.

Ferrante, E. A., Cudrici, C. D., & Boehm, M. (2019). CADASIL: New advances in basic science and clinical perspectives. *Current Opinion in Hematology*, **26**(3), 193.

Fierini, F. (2020). Mixed dementia: Neglected clinical entity or nosographic artifice? *Journal of the Neurological Sciences*, **410**, 116662.

Gorelick, P. B., Scuteri, A., Black, S. E., et al. (2011). Vascular contributions to cognitive impairment and dementia: a statement for healthcare professionals from the American Heart Association/American Stroke Association. *Stroke*, **42**(9), 2672–713.

Graham, N. L., Emery, T., & Hodges, J. R. (2004). Distinctive cognitive profiles in Alzheimer's disease and subcortical vascular dementia. *Journal of Neurology, Neurosurgery & Psychiatry*, **75**, 61–71.

Gräsel, E., Cameron, S., & Lehrl, S. (1990). What contribution can the Hachinski Ischemic Scale make to the differential diagnosis between multi-infarct dementia and primary degenerative dementia? *Archives of Gerontology and Geriatrics*, **11**(1), 63–75.

Hachinski, V. C., & Bowler, J. V. (1993). Vascular dementia. *Neurology*, **43**, 2159–60.

Hachinski, V. C., Iliff, L. D., Zilhka, E., et al. (1975). Cerebral blood flow in dementia. *Archives of Neurology*, **32**(9), 632–7.

Hachinski, V. C., Lassen, N. A., & Marshall, J. (1974). Multi-infarct dementia: A cause of mental deterioration in the elderly. *The Lancet*, **304**(7874), 207–9.

Hébert, R., & Brayne, C. (1995). Epidemiology of vascular dementia. *Neuroepidemiology*, **14**(5), 240–57.

Herbert, V., Brookes, R. L., Markus, H. S., & Morris, R. G. (2014). Verbal fluency in cerebral small vessel disease and Alzheimer's disease. *Journal of the International Neuropsychological Society*, **20**(4), 413–21.

Iadecola, C., Duering, M., Hachinski, V., et al. (2019). Vascular cognitive impairment and dementia: JACC scientific expert panel. *Journal of the American College of Cardiology*, **73**(25), 3326–44.

Jordan, F., Quinn, T. J., McGuinness, B., et al. (2020). Aspirin and other non-steroidal anti-inflammatory drugs for the prevention of dementia. *Cochrane Database of Systematic Reviews*, **4**, CD011459.

Jorm, A. F., & Jolley, D. (1998). The incidence of dementia: A meta-analysis. *Neurology*, **51**(3), 728–33.

Klohs, J. (2019). An integrated view on vascular dysfunction in Alzheimer's disease. *Neurodegenerative Diseases*, **19**(3–4), 109–27.

Knopman, D. S., DeKosky, S. T., Cummings, J. L., et al. (2001). Practice parameter: Diagnosis of dementia (an evidence-based review): Report of the Quality Standards Subcommittee of the American Academy of Neurology. *Neurology*, **56**(9), 1143–53.

Krishnan, K. R. (2002). Biological risk factors in late life depression. *Biological Psychiatry*, **52**, 185–92.

Kua, E. H., Ho, E., Tan, H. H., et al. (2014). The natural history of dementia. *Psychogeriatrics*, **14**(3), 196–201.

Moroney, J. T., Bagiella, E., Desmond, D. W., et al. (1997). Meta-analysis of the Hachinski Ischemic Score in pathologically verified dementias. *Neurology*, **49**(4), 1096–105.

Niwa, K., Kazama, K., Younkin, L., et al. (2002). Cerebrovascular autoregulation is profoundly impaired in mice overexpressing amyloid precursor protein. *American Journal of Physiology-Heart and Circulatory Physiology*, **283**(1), H315–H323.

O'Brien, J., & Thomas, A. (2015). Vascular dementia. *The Lancet*, **386**(10004), 1698–706.

Pendlebury, S. T., & Rothwell, P. M. (2009). Prevalence, incidence, and factors associated with pre-stroke and post-stroke dementia: A systematic review and meta-analysis. *The Lancet Neurology*, **8** (11), 1006–18.

Pendlebury, S. T., Wadling, S., Silver, L. E., Mehta, Z., & Rothwell, P. M. (2011). Transient cognitive impairment in TIA and minor stroke. *Stroke*, **42**(11), 3116–21.

Price, C. C., Jefferson, A. L., Merino, J. G., Heilman, K. M., & Libon, D. J. (2005). Subcortical vascular dementia: Integrating neuropsychological and neuroradiologic data. *Neurology*, **65**(3), 376–82.

Purnell, C., Gao, S., Callahan, C. M., & Hendrie, H. C. (2009). Cardiovascular risk factors and incident Alzheimer disease: A systematic review of the literature. *Alzheimer Disease and Associated Disorders*, **23**(1), 1–10.

Rasquin, S. M. C., Lodder, J., & Verhey, F. R. J. (2005). Predictors of reversible mild cognitive impairment after stroke: A 2-year follow-up study. *Journal of the Neurological Sciences*, **229**, 21–5.

Román, G. C. (2004). Facts, myths, and controversies in vascular dementia. *Journal of the Neurological Sciences*, **226**(1–2), 49–52.

Román, G. C., Tatemichi, T. K., Erkinjuntti, T., et al. (1993). Vascular dementia: diagnostic criteria for research studies: Report of the NINDS-AIREN International Workshop. *Neurology*, **43**(2), 250.

Sachdev, P. S., Brodaty, H., Valenzuela, M. J., et al. (2004). The neuropsychological profile of vascular cognitive impairment in stroke and TIA patients. *Neurology*, **62**(6), 912–19.

Sachdev, P., Kalaria, R., O'Brien, J., et al. (2014). Diagnostic criteria for vascular cognitive disorders: A VASCOG statement. *Alzheimer Disease and Associated Disorders*, **28**(3), 206–18.

Skrobot, O. A., Black, S. E., Chen, C., et al. (2018). Progress toward standardized diagnosis of vascular cognitive impairment: Guidelines from the Vascular Impairment of Cognition Classification Consensus Study. *Alzheimer's & Dementia*, **14**(3), 280–292.

Smith, E. E. (2017). Clinical presentations and epidemiology of vascular dementia. *Clinical Science*, **131**(11), 1059–68.

Snowden, D. (2001). *Aging with Grace: What the Nun Study Teaches Us About Leading Longer, Healthier and More Meaningful Lives.* New York: Bantam Press.

Snowdon, D. A., Greiner, L. H., Mortimer, et al. (1997). Brain infarction and the clinical expression of Alzheimer disease: The Nun Study. *JAMA*, **277**(10), 813–17.

Tiel, C., Sudo, F. K., Alves, G. S., et al. (2015). Neuropsychiatric symptoms in vascular cognitive impairment: a systematic review. *Dementia & Neuropsychologia*, **9**, 230–6.

Tierney, M. C., Black, S. E., Szalai, J. P., et al. (2001). Recognition memory and verbal fluency differentiate probable Alzheimer disease from subcortical ischemic vascular dementia. *Archives of Neurology*, **58**(10), 1654–9.

Toledo, J. B., Arnold, S. E., Raible, K., et al. (2013). Contribution of cerebrovascular disease in autopsy confirmed neurodegenerative disease cases in the National Alzheimer's Coordinating Centre. *Brain*, **136**(9), 2697–706.

Traykov, L., Baudic, S., Raoux, N., et al. (2005). Patterns of memory impairment and perseverative behavior discriminate early Alzheimer's disease from subcortical vascular dementia. *Journal of the Neurological Sciences*, **229**, 75–9.

Vasquez, B. P., & Zakzanis, K. K. (2015). The neuropsychological profile of vascular cognitive impairment not demented: A meta-analysis. *Journal of Neuropsychology*, **9**(1), 109–36.

Wen, W., Sachdev, P. S., Li, J. J., Chen, X., & Anstey, K. J. (2009). White matter hyperintensities in the forties: Their prevalence and topography in an epidemiological sample aged 44–48. *Human Brain Mapping*, **30**(4), 1155–67.

Wolters, F. J., & Ikram, M. A. (2019). Epidemiology of vascular dementia: Nosology in a time of epiomics. *Arteriosclerosis, Thrombosis, and Vascular Biology*, **39**(8), 1542–9.

Yoshitake, T., Kiyohara, Y., Kato, I., et al. (1995). Incidence and risk factors of vascular dementia and Alzheimer's disease in a defined elderly Japanese population: The Hisayama Study. *Neurology*, **45**(6), 1161–8.

Zekry, D., Duyckaerts, C., Moulias, R., et al. (2002). Degenerative and vascular lesions of the brain have synergistic effects in dementia of the elderly. *Acta Neuropathologica*, **103**(5), 481–7.

Lewy Body Dementia, Parkinson's Disease and Parkinson's Dementia, and Parkinson's Plus

This chapter deals with a series of highly inter-related disorders, which are linked by a common toxic agent: the Lewy body. These are accumulations of an insoluble form of alpha-synuclein protein, and are found in Parkinson's disease, Parkinson's dementia, dementia with Lewy bodies (DLB) and multiple systems atrophy (MSA) (Gomperts, 2016). Although these disorders share a common proteinopathy, their clinical presentations differ as a result of the distribution of this protein throughout the brain. Two further syndromes – progressive supranuclear palsy (PSP) and corticobasal degeneration (CBD) – are also classified as Parkinsonian disorders, but are associated with abnormal tau protein rather than alpha-synuclein (Kouri et al., 2011; Stanford et al., 2000).

Whilst patients with possible Parkinson's dementia may present at memory clinics, diagnosis of Parkinson's disease is usually done within more specialist clinics run by neurologists or geriatricians as it initially presents as a movement disorder.

Parkinson's Disease

Prevalence

Approximately 70% of cases of Parkinsonism are caused by Parkinson's disease (PD) (Benito-León et al., 2003). Parkinson's UK reported the prevalence of PD in the UK as 286.5 per 100,000, with an incidence of 33.4 per 100,000 person years (Parkinson's UK, 2018). The prevalence rate increases with age, and almost doubles every five years between the ages of 50–69 for both men and women. The disorder is more common in men, with a ratio of 1:1.5 reported for the age ranges of 50–89.

Pathology

Some of the mechanisms of PD have been well understood for many years now, particularly surrounding the role of the neurotransmitter dopamine, which led to the development of pharmacological and surgical treatments (Jankovic & Aguilar, 2008). The progression of the disease is also well understood, largely thanks to post-mortem brain bank studies (Braak et al., 2003). The motor signs of the disease are associated with degeneration of an area in the mid-brain called the substantia nigra, which produces the neurotransmitter dopamine. Normal function appears to be possible until more than 75% of the cells in that region have degenerated, at which point there is insufficient dopamine available to supply the basal ganglia. This sets off a chain of imbalanced inhibitory and excitatory signals in the various structures between the basal ganglia and the motor cortex in the frontal lobes, resulting in a loss of motor control which manifests as slowing and tremors.

The time course of PD is very long, with Lewy bodies accumulating for many years before any clinical signs become apparent. Braak et al. (2003) described the progression of Lewy bodies as starting in the dorsal motor nucleus of the vagus nerve and olfactory bulb, before moving to the brainstem, mid-brain, and substantia nigra. In the final stages Lewy bodies are found in the diencephalon and cortex. There are reports of symptoms such as constipation, sleep disorders, mood disorders, loss of smell, and heart arrhythmias in patients with PD, which can pre-date the development of movement disorders by some years (Morens et al., 1996). Age of onset appears related to rate of progression, with young onset being characterised by a slower progression, and a rapid progression being associated with late onset (Van Rooden et al., 2010). There have been a number of suggestions for different subtypes, although there is no consensus on this at present (Postuma et al., 2016).

A further intriguing suggestion is that the spread of Lewy bodies can operate as an infective process as you can get transmission of Lewy bodies between species, which so there may be cases where it resembles a form of prion disorder (Iansek & Dandoudis, 2019), spreading to the vagus nerve via the gut.

Diagnostic Criteria for PD

Whilst diagnosis of PD is likely to occur via a movement disorders clinic, rather than a memory clinic, the criteria for PD are briefly discussed here. Movement problems remain core for diagnosis, but the criteria were revised to take account of the increased recognition of non-motor signs which can often occur at early stages in the disease (Postuma et al., 2015). There are also criteria for prodromal PD (Berg et al., 2015). The Movement Disorders Society diagnostic criteria (Postuma et al., 2015) retain the centrality of movement disorder, by first considering whether Parkinsonism is present, which is bradykinesia (slowed movements) combined with rigidity, resting tremor, or both. If present, the question is addressed of whether this is due to PD by looking for (a) absolute exclusion criteria (e.g. cortical sensory loss, downward gaze palsy), (b) red flags such as rapid progression of gait abnormality requiring a wheelchair within five years, and/or absence of common non-motor features after five years, and (c) supportive criteria which relates to a significant and unequivocal response to dopaminergic therapy. Two levels of certainty are employed. Clinically established PD requires absence of absolute exclusion criteria, at least two supportive criteria, and no red flags. Clinically probable PD requires there to be no absolute exclusion criteria and red flags counterbalanced by supportive criteria (i.e. one supportive feature per red flag), up to a maximum of two red flags.

Biomarkers (other than imaging) do not feature in the Parkinson's diagnostic criteria as there is currently no marker to identify alpha-synuclein protein.

Cognitive Changes with Parkinson's Disease

It has long been recognised that PD patients without dementia may still experience cognitive decline. Pirozzolo et al. (1982) reported that cognitive deficits were apparent in 96% of patients when compared to controls. Deficits were mainly reported in visuospatial tasks, memory, and executive function. Dubois and Pillon (1997) questioned whether the widely reported visual-spatial deficits may actually arise because those tasks are more cognitively demanding and focussed on the executive deficits as primary. Part of their reasoning was that deficits are apparent on more demanding visual-spatial tasks (e.g. set-shifting), and are likely to result from the interplay between circuits of the basal ganglia and those of the frontal lobes. Although the basal ganglia are involved in a number of functions, Wu, Kansuku, and Hallet (2004) considered that the role of the basal ganglia in all functions is to automate performance of tasks, so they rely less on attentional resources. With this function impaired, patients with PD must devote more attentional resources to carrying out tasks which were previously automated.

Parkinsons disease dementia has been classified as a subcortical dementia (along with Huntington's disease), which is associated with a cognitive profile of deficits in executive function, speed of information processing, and working memory, but relative preservation of episodic memory and language (Pillon et al., 1993). However, in their systematic review of the literature, Litvan et al. (2011) cited a number of papers which collectively reported deficits in most aspects of cognitive function.

Parkinson's Disease Mild Cognitive Impairment

In line with the thinking on many cognitive disorders, criteria for mild cognitive impairment have been applied to Parkinson's disease (PD-MCI). In a systematic literature review, Litvan et al. (2011) reported that 26.7% of PD patients without dementia had PD-MCI, with a range of 18.9–38.2%. Non-amnestic single domain MCI was the most common form, and development of PD-MCI was associated with increasing age, disease duration, and disease severity. Cammisuli et al. (2019) also reported a relationship with age, as well as male gender and lower levels of education. A relationship with sleep disorders, daytime sleepiness, autonomic nervous system dysfunction, and mood disorders such as depression and anxiety has also been found (Palavra, Naismith, & Lewis, 2013). Janvin et al. (2006) reported 62% of patients with PD-MCI developed Parkinson's disease dementia (PDD) over a four-year period, compared with 20% of cognitively normal PD patients. Litvan et al. (2012) reported that progression to PDD is associated with non-amnestic single-domain MCI, executive deficits, impaired verbal fluency, visuospatial deficits, and memory and language dysfunction. Williams-Gray et al. (2009) followed up 126 patients over five years, finding that baseline measures of age ≥72 years, semantic fluency less than 20 words in 90 seconds, and inability to copy an intersecting pentagons figure were significant predictors of dementia risk.

Criteria for PD-MCI are based on the Petersen criteria (latest revision Albert et al., 2011), with the additional requirement for a diagnosis of PD and the addition of two levels according to the extent of neuropsychological assessment which has taken place (Litvan, 2011, 2012). Inclusion and exclusion criteria are summarised in Table 7.1.

Levels 1 and 2 are based on the extent of neuropsychological/cognitive testing which has taken place and are somewhat more explicit than the general recommendations for MCI (Albert at al., 2011). The PD-MCI criteria specify that assessment should cover five areas of cognitive function, carried over from the PDD criteria (Emre et al., 2007): attention/working memory, executive function, language, memory, and visuospatial abilities. Interestingly, speed of information processing is not included, as most methods of assessing this are usually based around psychomotor speed and would therefore be sensitive to motor slowing.

Level 1 is designated as 'abbreviated assessment/possible PD-MCI' and is based upon the use of global/screening instruments such as the MoCA or ACE. Alternatively, it may be based upon a 'limited' neuropsychological assessment which includes only one test of each aspect of cognitive function, or less than the full five specified cognitive domains. Although

Table 7.1 Diagnostic criteria for PD-MCI, based upon Litvan et al. (2012)

Inclusion criteria

Diagnosis of Parkinson's disease as based on the UK PD Brain Bank Criteria (Gibb & Lees, 1988)

Insidious cognitive decline caused primarily by the underlying disease process

Cognitive decline reported by either the patient or informant, or observed by the clinician

Deficits should be evident on cognitive testing, but should not interfere significantly with functional independence

Exclusion criteria

Diagnosis of PDD based on MDS taskforce criteria (Emre et al., 2007)

Other diagnoses may account for the cognitive decline (e.g. delirium, stroke, traumatic brain injury, medication)

Other PD-associated factors may impact upon cognitive testing (e.g. motor problems, sleepiness/fatigue, psychosis, severe anxiety)

Litvan et al. also recommend the use of a tool for estimating premorbid ability, such as the National Adult Reading Test (NART) (Nelson, 1982), it is difficult to see how this could be incorporated as global/screening instruments are typically based around a cut-off score rather than giving an ability range (see Chapters 2 and 4 for further discussion of this issue).

Level 2 is referred to as 'comprehensive assessment' and requires a formal neuropsychological assessment featuring at least two tests of each of the specified cognitive domains. Impairment should be present on at least two tests, either within a single cognitive domain or across different cognitive domains. Litvan et al. (2012) also specify the criteria to be used for impairment, which again goes slightly beyond that specified for general MCI (Albert et al., 2011). These are (1) performance one to two standard deviations lower than age, education, gender, and culturally appropriate norms, (2) significant decline on serial assessment (at least one standard deviation or exceeding the reliable change index), or (3) significant decline from estimated premorbid levels. The challenges involved in operationalising such criteria are discussed in Chapters 2 and 4 of this book.

Specification of the subtype of PD-MCI is only possible following a comprehensive assessment, and again differs slightly from the standard MCI classification of Albert et al. (2011). Single domain MCI is defined by having two abnormal tests within the same cognitive domain, and at least one abnormal test within two or more cognitive domains represents multiple domain MCI. However, Litvan et al. (2012) recommended specifying in which domains impairment was detected rather than using the amnestic/non-amnestic classification outlined in Albert et al. (2011).

Parkinson's Disease Dementia and Dementia with Lewy Bodies

There is a lack of consensus regarding whether PDD and DLB are different manifestations of the same disorder or separate entities. DSM-V classifies them as separate disorders, and gives separate diagnostic criteria. Another way to consider them is that they sit on a spectrum of cognitive severity, with PD and PDD at the mild end, DLB in the middle, and DLB with Alzheimer's at the severe end (Jellinger, 2018). They share a common toxic agent, along with MSA, in the form of alpha-synuclein protein accumulating within neurons, and they both require the presence of Parkinsonism. The distribution of Lewy bodies is different, as is order of onset of symptoms (Emre et al., 2007). The key difference clinically is (a) if Parkinsonian motor signs have been present for at least a year prior to the onset of dementia, the diagnosis is PDD; (b) if the onset of motor signs is within a year prior to the onset of dementia, or up to a year after the onset of dementia, the diagnosis is DLB (Emre et al., 2007). The updated criteria for DLB state that DLB should be diagnosed if cognitive problems develop before or concurrent with motor symptoms (McKeith et al., 2017). Note that for a diagnosis of DLB, Parkinsonian motor signs *should* be apparent within a year of developing dementia, although some studies have suggested that up to 25% of DLB patients may not develop motor signs (Kim, Kågedal, & Halliday, 2014). Once Parkinsonism is present, PDD and DLB cannot be distinguished clinically or pathologically (Friedman, 2017).

We will first consider PDD, including diagnostic criteria, then focus on DLB and consider the differences between them, before moving onto the relationship with Alzheimer's disease.

Parkinson's Disease Dementia

Prevalence and Incidence

Cummings (1988) originally estimated the prevalence rate of dementia within the PD population to be around 40%, although this did not differentiate between PDD and DLB. Other prevalence rates within PD populations have varied from 22% (De Lau et al., 2005) to 48% (Hobson & Meara, 2004). Hely et al. (2005) carried out a 15-year follow-up study of patients with PD and reported 48% had dementia, 36% had MCI, and 15% were cognitively normal. Aarsland, Zaccai, and Brayne (2005) carried out a systematic literature review which suggested that 24–31% of patients with PD have PDD. This represents 3.6% of cases of dementia as a whole, and 0.2–0.5% of the general population over 65.

Roughly 10% of the PD population develop dementia each year (Emre et al., 2007), and 50% of patients with PD are likely to develop dementia within 10 years of diagnosis (Williams-Gray et al., 2013). People with PD are 3.5 times more likely to develop dementia than the general population (Yip, Brayne, & Mathews, 2006). There is a similar gender distribution in PD and PDD reported in the literature, with a male-to-female ratio of roughly 2:1 (Mouton et al., 2018).

Factors Which Predict Development of PDD

Several longitudinal studies have been carried out which looked at PD patients without dementia at baseline and considered which characteristic predicted who would develop dementia.

Hughes et al. (2000) reported that age at entry into the study and severity of motor symptoms predicted dementia; age at disease onset and disease duration did not. Williams-Gray et al. (2009) carried out a 5-year longitudinal study with 126 patients with PD. They found the factors which predicted development of PDD over that time period were age over 71 years, a semantic fluency score of less than 20 words in 90 seconds, and an inability to copy intersecting pentagons. Phonemic fluency and other frontally based tasks were not predictive of developing PDD. Anang et al. (2014) reported that cardiovascular problems, poor colour discrimination, and gait disturbance were all predictive, but the biggest predictor was the presence/absence of REM sleep disorder. Phongpreecha et al. (2020) looked at biological and cognitive factors, reporting that age, disease duration, sex, and the presence of the glucocerebrosidase gene were the most predictive biological factors. The presence of APOE ε4 was not an overall predictive factor, but, rather, more specifically predicted a reduction in semantic fluency for women. However, biological factors were less predictive than the cognitive factors, with MoCA overall score, semantic fluency, digit symbol, and trail making being the strongest predictors of developing PDD.

Cognitive Profile Associated with PDD

Aldridge et al. (2018) compared a battery of neuropsychological tests in patients with PDD and DLB, reporting no significant differences in cognitive profile (i.e. they were not able to distinguish between the two groups on the basis of neuropsychological test scores). This was consistent with several previous papers which found no cognitive differences between the two clinical groups (Downes et al., 1998; Gnanalingham et al., 1997; Mosimann et al., 2004). Although one study reported DLB patients performing worse on verbal memory (Filoteo et al., 2009), this study also found that a number of the participants also had comorbid Alzheimer's disease at post-mortem examination or had originally been diagnosed as DAT. Janvin et al. (2006) suggested that there are two distinct cognitive profiles, although they occur with roughly equal frequency in both PDD and DLB. These are (1) a subcortical profile, characterised by deficits in executive function (initiation and perseveration), attention, and visuospatial construction, which was seen in 56% of PDD patients and 55% of DLB patients, and (2) a cortical profile characterised by memory impairments which was seen in 30% of PDD patients and 26% of DLB patients. By contrast, the cortical profile was seen in 67% of patients with DAT. However, it should be noted that DAT and PD can co-occur, so a cortical profile may in some cases arise from DAT pathology.

In general, the primary cognitive deficits in PDD are considered to be attention and executive function, with relatively preserved memory. In DAT, the primary deficits are verbal memory and delayed memory, with executive function and attention being less affected (Vasconcellos & Pereira, 2015). These differences are more likely to be apparent in the early stages of the disease, as with all dementias the relatively preserved aspects of cognition also decline as the disease progresses.

Mood Disorders

Hallucinations and, to a lesser extent, delusions are found in both PDD and DLB. Anxiety and depression are also common, which may be caused directly by the disease process or indirectly as a response to changes brought about by the disease. Aarsland et al. (2001) reported relative rates of major depression within a community-based study as 9% for PD, 13% for PDD, and 19% for DLB. Anxiety appears to present with a similar frequency to depression (Emre et al., 2007).

Diagnostic Criteria for PDD

The Movement Disorders Society published diagnostic criteria for PDD (Emre et al., 2007) to describe dementia which occurs in the context of 'well-established' PD, distinguishing between probable and possible PDD.

A diagnosis of probable PDD requires:

1. Core features: the presence of a diagnosis of both (a) PD and (b) dementia with a gradual development within the context of established PD.
2. Associated clinical features: (a) Typical cognitive profile with deficits in two out of four core areas (attention, executive function, visuospatial processing, and free recall which improves with cueing); (b) at least one behavioural symptom (apathy, anxiety, depression, hallucinations, delusions). However, a diagnosis can still be made in the absence of behavioural symptoms.
3. An absence of features which make the diagnosis uncertain. These are defined as (a) other abnormalities which may give rise to cognitive impairment although not thought to be the cause of dementia (e.g. vascular disease identified on imaging), or (b) the time interval between development of cognitive and motor symptoms being unknown.
4. Absence of (a) other conditions which may impact upon cognition, such as delirium or major depression, and (b) features compatible with probable vascular dementia.

Possible PDD requires the presence of both core features, and the absence of delirium, major depression, or features compatible with vascular dementia. However, it allows for (a) an atypical cognitive profile, which might include aphasia or 'storage failure amnesia', in the absence of an attention deficit, and/or an absence of behavioural symptoms, and (b) features which make the diagnosis uncertain (such as evidence of vascular pathology on imaging) and unknown time interval between development of cognitive and motor problems.

Dementia with Lewy Bodies

Having stated that the only reliable clinical distinction between PDD and DLB is the order in which motor and cognitive symptoms occur, DLB still deserves individual consideration as this is more likely to present within the context of a memory assessment service and has separate diagnostic criteria. When someone presents for cognitive assessment, Parkinsonism may not yet have developed, therefore more weighting must be placed on other features to distinguish DLB from other forms of dementia such as DAT.

Prevalence and Incidence

DLB is considered to be the second most common form of degenerative dementia after DAT (McKeith et al., 2004), although the prevalence rates cited in different studies vary considerably. Zaccai, McCracken, and Brayne (2005) carried out a systematic review of prevalence and incidence studies and reported prevalence rates ranging from 0 to 5% of the general population aged over 65, and 0–30.5% of dementia cases. At that time only one incidence study was available, which gave an incidence rate of 0.1% for the general population, and 3.2% per year for new dementia cases. A later review concluded that DLB accounts for roughly 5% of dementia cases in adults over the age of 65, with incidence rates of 3.2–7.1% of all dementia cases (Hogan et al., 2016).

Age of Onset and Progression

Age of onset has been reported as 50–70 (Schoenberg & Duff, 2011). Earlier onset has been reported; for example, Takao et al. (2004) reported a case where cognitive problems were first noted at age 13, progressing rapidly to death at age 15. The life expectancy of someone with DLB is typically 7.3 years (Williams et al., 2006), although a rapid-onset variant (rpDLB) has been described with a mean duration of 9 months (Gaig et al., 2011).

Sleep Disorders in DLB

Sleep disorders, in particular REM sleep disorder, have been widely reported in the development of Lewy body disorders. Chan et al. (2018) reported that 38–65% of patients with REM sleep disorder developed either PD, MSA, or DLB 10–20 years after initial presentation. However, REM sleep disorder has become particularly associated with DLB to the extent that it is now considered a core clinical feature in the updated diagnostic criteria (McKeith et al., 2017). Salthouse, Bradshaw, and Sailing (2019) reviewed the literature on sleep disturbances in DLB, particularly electrophysiological (EEG) evidence, and concluded that DLB is characterised by a loss of boundaries between (1) different sleep states, and (2) intermittent loss of the distinction between sleep and waking. It has also been suggested that hallucinations in DLB may represent elements of REM sleep intruding into wakefulness (Nomura et al., 2003).

Diagnostic Criteria for DLB

The DLB consortium updated the diagnostic criteria in 2017 (McKeith et al., 2017). There must be evidence of dementia, as in a gradual decline in cognitive abilities which interferes with everyday function. A decline in memory may not be apparent until the later stages of the disease, whereas attention, visuospatial, and executive problems may be seen relatively early. The core clinical features of DLB are:

1. Hallucinations
2. Fluctuations in cognition (both during the day, and between different days)
3. Parkinsonism
4. REM sleep disorder

Supportive clinical features are listed as severe sensitivity to antipsychotic agents, postural instability, repeated falls, syncope or other transient episodes of unresponsiveness, and severe autonomic dysfunction.

The criteria also include use of biomarkers. Indicative biomarkers are specified as (a) reduced dopamine transporter uptake (DAT) in the basal ganglia demonstrated by SPECT or PET, (b) abnormal (low uptake)[123] iodine MIBG myocardial scintigraphy, or (c) polysomnographic confirmation of REM sleep without atonia. Supportive biomarkers are specified as (a) relative preservation of medial temporal lobe structures on CT/MRI scan, (b) generalised low uptake on SPECT/PET perfusion/metabolism scan with reduced occipital activity in the cingulate island sign on FDG-PET imaging, and (c) prominent posterior slow-wave activity on EEG with periodic fluctuations in the pre-alpha/theta range.

A diagnosis of *probable* DLB can be made if two or more core clinical features are present, or if one core clinical feature is present accompanied by one or more indicative biomarker(s). A diagnosis of *possible* DLB can be made based on one core feature without evidence from biomarkers, or one or more indicative biomarker(s) even if no core features are present.

A DLB diagnosis is less likely if there is other disease which could account for the clinical presentation, either in part or in total (e.g. cerebrovascular disease). Although this may indicate a mixed picture rather than excluding DLB. It is also less likely if Parkinsonism is the only core feature and presents at a relatively advanced stage of dementia.

A DLB diagnosis requires dementia to present before or concurrently with motor symptoms.

Hallucinations, Confabulations, and Charles Bonnet Syndrome

Some care needs to be taken when considering the presence of hallucinations during the diagnostic process. Hallucinations can appear in the advanced stages of most dementias, which is one of many reasons to assess people in as early a stage of the disease as possible. It is also important to consider whether reported hallucinations may in fact be confabulations, which can present when both memory and executive function are impaired (as in Wenicke–Korsakoff syndrome). The difference is that an hallucination is a perception of something which is not there, whereas a confabulation is a false memory. For example, if someone states they can see a horse in the corner of the room which nobody else can see, this is likely to be a hallucination. If they report there had been a horse in the room earlier, this may be a confabulation. Hallucinations early in the disease process are a hallmark of DLB, whereas confabulations are not.

Another disorder of which to be aware is Charles Bonnet syndrome (CBS), in which hallucinations arise in the context of visual impairment such as macular degeneration, usually unaccompanied by cognitive deficits. Although the hallucinations can be vivid and well-formed, people with CBS are usually aware that these perceptions are not real (Shadlu, Shadlu, & Shepherd, 2009). Hallucinations in DLB are vivid and well-formed, but crucially occur within the context of cognitive decline without impairment in basic visual processes. It is also relatively common for patients with DLB to interact with their hallucinations (Mosiman et al., 2004). It is of course possible for someone with visual impairment to develop DLB, as the two disorders may co-occur.

DLB-MCI

Although there are not separate criteria for DLB-MCI, a number of studies have been conducted applying standard MCI criteria (Albert et al., 2011). When compared to patients with Alzheimer-related MCI, DLB-MCI patients tend to perform worse on visuospatial and letter fluency tasks, but better on memory tasks (Sadiq et al., 2017).

A Comparison of PDD and DLB

Although for diagnostic purposes the key difference between PDD and DLB is whether cognitive deficits appeared after the development of Parkinsonism, or concurrent with/after it, there are some differences between the two disorders, some of which are summarised in Table 7.2. These are patterns reported in group comparisons, but they represent relative frequencies and are not absolutes upon which to base a differential diagnosis.

Comorbidity with Alzheimer's Pathology

Although PD, PDD, and DLB are considered to be caused by an accumulation of alpha-synuclein protein in the form of Lewy bodies, post-mortem studies have consistently identified the presence of amyloid and tau proteins, which are the hallmarks of Alzheimers's disease (Jellinger, 2018). AD pathology appears to be more significant in DLB than PDD (Walker, Stefanis, & Attems, 2019), with biomarker studies indicating that around 50% of DLB patients also have AD pathology (Ossenkoppele et al.,

Table 7.2 Comparison of some features of PDD and DLB

Feature	PDD	DLB	Reference
Hallucinations	54% of patients experience these, but often in relation to medications	76% of patients experience these spontaneously, and they are considered a core feature	Aarsland et al. (2001)
Interaction with hallucinations	Less likely to be actively involved	Frequently react to and interact	Mosiman et al. (2004)
Severe neuroleptic sensitivity	Reported in 39% of patients	Reported in 53% of patients	Aarsland et al. (2005)
REM sleep disorder	25–58% of patients	90% of patients and considered to be a core feature	Hu (2020)
Fluctuations in cognition	8.9% of patients	25% of patients and considered to be a core feature	Savica et al. (2013)
Delusions	Seen in 29% of patients	Seen in 57% of patients, can arise in later stages of the disease	Aarsland et al. (2001)
Presence of beta amyloid protein	Less common	Higher burden in the neocortex and striatum	Ruffman et al. (2016)

2015). Although the extent of AD pathology may not be extensive in all cases, cases of pure Lewy body pathology may be relatively rare (Gurd et al., 2000). Lewy body burden in the cortex appears to be an independent predictor of developing dementia, although the greater the burden of beta amyloid protein the more rapid the cognitive decline (Ruffman et al., 2016). The presence of AD pathology in addition to alpha-synuclein results in a more severe manifestation of the disease, with the cumulative burden of the different proteins collectively adding to cognitive decline (Walker, Stefanis, & Attems, 2019).

Alpha-synuclein has also been observed in the brains of people with a primary diagnosis of DAT, although it tends to accumulate in the cell bodies, whereas with PD it is more commonly seen in the axons and dendrites (Kim, Kågedal, & Halliday, 2014).

Genetics

PDD and DLB are considered to be largely sporadic, and there are no sufficiently strong genetic factors to be diagnostic (Jellinger, 2018). However, an increased risk has been identified in connection with the APOE4 gene and DLB, and to a lesser extent with PDD (Vergow et al., 2017). Another gene, glucocerebrosidase (GBA) has also been associated with an increased risk of PDD (Brockman et al., 2015) and DLB (Nalls et al., 2013).

Response to Medication

One of the causal mechanisms in Parkinsonism is under-production of the neurotransmitter dopamine as a result of the loss of cells in the mid-brain which produce it. PD, PDD, and DLB all show a good response to treatment with L-Dopa (Bonelli et al., 2004). Although this is not a disease-modifying treatment, it can bring about a reduction in Parkinsonian motor problems. Its effect on cognition is more variable, with both positive and negative effects being reported (Cools, 2006). A lack of response to L-Dopa is one factor which can be indictive of an atypical Parkinsonian presentation.

Atypical Parkinsonian Disorders

These are a collection of disorders which show Parkinsonian features but are not classified as forms of PD. Originally referred to as Parkinson's plus, they are now more commonly referred to as atypical Parkinsonian syndromes and consist of MSA, PSP, and corticobasal degeneration, and collectively account for up to 20% of Parkinsonian presentations (Potashkin et al., 2012). These disorders tend not to respond well to treatment with L-Dopa (Moretti, 2019). They will only briefly be considered here, as they are likely to be diagnosed in the context of a movement disorder clinic rather than a memory assessment service.

Multiple System Atrophy

MSA is a rapidly progressing Parkinsonian disorder which is diagnosed primarily on the basis of autonomic dysfunction, Parkinsonism, and cerebellar dysfunction (Wenning et al., 2022). Cognitive changes are not considered diagnostic, even though they may be present.

The toxic agent in MSA is alpha-synuclein, which it has in common with PD and DLB, but the clinical presentation differs. Although there is evidence for a decline in cognitive ability, it usually does not meet the criteria for dementia (Kao et al., 2009) and a change in cognitive ability is not included in the diagnostic criteria (Wenning et al., 2022). Dementia developing within three years of symptom onset is an exclusion criteria for this diagnosis. MSA differs from PDD and BLB in the way alpha-synuclein accumulates as it is found predominantly in the oligodendrocytes of the cerebellum and brainstem rather than within neurons (Kim et al., 2014), and these deposits are known as glial cytoplasmic inclusions rather than Lewy bodies. Neuronal loss predominantly occurs in striatonigral and olivopontocerebellar systems (Wenning et al., 2022). Average age of onset has been reported as 54.2 years, with an average survival of 6.2 years (Ben-Schlomo et al., 1997). Late-onset cases are rare and have been reported to have a poorer prognosis, with a median survival time of 3 years and more pronounced cognitive impairment (Sekiya et al., 2022).

The cognitive decline seen in MSA is mainly in executive function, although memory and visuospatial processing can also be impaired (Stankovic et al., 2014). A reduced speed of information processing has also been reported (Koga et al., 2017), although this can be hard to measure if there is also motor slowing. It was noted that the cognitive deficits were more likely to be detected by a more extensive neuropsychology assessment than via cognitive screens. Depression and anxiety are common, but not hallucinations (Kao et al., 2009).

Progressive Supranuclear Palsy

PSP is a degenerative disorder with Parkinsonian symptoms, but unlike the disorders considered so far in this chapter, it is a tauopathy rather than a synucleinopathy. Unlike MSA, it can present with marked cognitive decline at a relatively early stage so neuropsychological assessment may play a useful role in the diagnostic process and has been included in the diagnostic criteria, which is made on the basis of four factors: oculomotor dysfunction, postural instability, akinesia, and cognitive dysfunction (Höglinger et al., 2017). PSP has different subtypes, with the most common form being Richardson's syndrome, characterised by postural instability, falls, and inability to move the eyes deliberately in a vertical motion (vertical supranuclear gaze palsy) (Höglinger et al., 2017). Average age of onset has been reported as 63, with a mean survival time of 5 years (Litvan et al., 1996). Initial presenting signs are usually postural instability and falls, including backwards falls, and visual problems (Nath et al., 2003). Cognitively, PSP presents in a similar manner to frontotemporal dementia (FTD). Lagarde et al. (2013) compared patients with the Richardson form of PSP to patients with behavioural variant FTD and concluded the cognitive profiles and pattern of atrophy were similar. The negative behavioural signs of FTD (apathy, aspontaneity, and indifference) are more common than the positive signs (irritability, social inappropriateness, impulsivity) (Gerstenecker, 2017).

Corticobasal Degeneration

Like PSP, CBD is also a tauopathy, with accumulation of hyperphosphorylated tau in both neurons and glial cells (Dickson et al., 2002). It is characterised by the development of motor problems usually affecting one side only, and higher cortical functions including apraxia, alien limb phenomena, cortical sensory loss, cognitive impairment, aphasia, and behavioural changes (Armstrong et al., 2013). Average age of onset is 63, and average life expectancy is 7 years (Wenning et al., 1998). CBD can have a varied presentation, which has led to five phenotypes being proposed, two of which (probable cortical-basal syndrome and possible corticobasal syndrome) are not based on cognitive change and two of which parallel types of FTD (frontal behavioural spatial syndrome and non-fluent/agrammatic variant of primary progressive aphasia). A final phenotype resembles PSP (Armstrong et al., 2013).

The Role of Imaging Data in PDD, DLB, and Atypical Parkinsonian Syndromes

Diagnosis of Parkinsonian syndromes is still clinically based, and neuroimaging techniques have traditionally not been recommended for use in routine clinical practice (Pagano, Niccolini, & Politis, 2016). However, the revised criteria for diagnosing DLB (McKeith et al., 2017) introduced some biomarkers under the headings of indicative and supportive, rather than core features. At the time of writing no biomarkers had been developed to directly identify alpha-synuclein pathology. There is some evidence that structural MRI can be useful in differential diagnosis of Parkinsonian disorders (e.g. asymmetric atrophy in frontal and parietal lobes supporting CBD) (Gallagher, 2019), with relative preservation of medial temporal lobe structures in DLB (McKeith et al., 2017). However, this is complicated by the heterogeneity of different Parkinsonian disorders, as some can result in a similar pattern of atrophy. There are certain hallmarks associated with particular disorders, such as a cruciform pontine hyperintensity (hot cross bun sign) in the cerebellar subtype of MSA, and atrophy of the mid-brain when compared to the pons in PSP, known as the 'hummingbird' sign (Saeed et al., 2020). The use of dopamine transport scans (DaT scan) using single-photon emission CT (SPECT) has proven useful for distinguishing genuine Parkinsonian disorders from other disorders such as Alzheimer's disease and vascular Parkinsonism, but is less effective at distinguishing PD from atypical Parkinsonian syndromes (Pagano, Niccolini, & Politis, 2016).

There is a great deal of research being conducted into the use of biomarkers, and most likely there is potential for distinguishing between the different types of Parkinsonian syndromes, where different pathologies can underlie similar presentations. However, there is usually a considerable delay before new technologies become available in clinical practice, and diagnoses based upon clinical presentation are likely to remain common practice for some time.

Key Points

- The Parkinsonian syndromes are a collection of degenerative brain diseases which affect movement and cognitive function. They are also associated with neuropsychiatric signs such as hallucinations (in PD and DLB), depression, and anxiety.
- Parkinson's disease accounts for roughly 70% of Parkinsonian presentations, and typically leads to dementia (PDD) after a number of years.
- DLB is related to PDD, but the cognitive problems develop either before or at the same time as the motor signs. Once the motor signs have developed, DLB and PDD are very similar.
- DLB has a very distinctive presentation, with four core features: hallucinations, fluctuations, Parkinsonian signs, and REM sleep disorder.
- Both PDD and DLB primarily affect executive function, attention, and visuospatial processing. Memory is relatively well-preserved.
- In PDD and DLB the toxic agent is an accumulation of alpha-synuclein protein which forms in clumps called Lewy bodies.
- Post-mortem examinations have shown the presence of Alzheimer-type pathology in DLB and to a lesser extent in PDD. It is therefore possible that the cognitive deficits observed may represent the cumulative effects of both pathologies.
- There are three recognised atypical Parkinsonian syndromes: MSA, PSP, and CBD. They are distinguished from PD by a poor response to treatment with L-Dopa.
- MSA is also caused by accumulation of alpha-synuclein, typically within the glial cells rather than within the neurons. These are known as glial cytoplasmic inclusions rather that Lewy bodies. Patients with MSA often have cognitive impairment, but rarely dementia.
- PSP and CBD are related to accumulation of tau protein. Dementia is more common with these syndromes than with MSA. The atypical Parkinsonian syndromes have a number of different subtypes, and can vary greatly in their presentations.

Appendix H   Case Studies

Case Study: VW

VW was a 67-year-old male who was referred via his GP with 'memory' problems, mood swings, and visual hallucinations. At the time of presentation, there were no reports of motor problems, although when VW attended for his neuropsychological assessment it was noted that he walked with a shuffling gait. His partner reported this was a recent development and had not been present when he was seen for her screening assessment. A clear example of REM sleep disorder was not reported; however, VW's partner considered the hallucinations to occur mainly on waking. In particular, he appeared to wake from a dream, but continued to experience elements of the dream whilst awake and interacted with characters from the dream. There were other examples of visual hallucinations when waking during the night, although they usually disappeared when he put the light on. These had increased in frequency over the last 18 months. VW's neuropsychological assessment indicated deficits in executive function and attention of more than two standard deviations. Memory scores were between 1 and 1.5 standard deviations lower than expected. His partner reported that his cognition fluctuated, with good days and bad days. A CT scan revealed no abnormalities, but a DaTscan reported reduced dopamine uptake. A diagnosis of probable DLB was arrived at on the basis of hallucinations, fluctuating cognition, recent development of a shuffling gait, and a DaTscan result consistent with DLB.

Case Study: BF

BF was a 70-year-old male who had been diagnosed with PD five years previously. BF reported increased difficulty with concentration and found it difficult to read novels, which he had previously enjoyed doing. He also reported some low mood, which had developed since the onset of his diagnosis. He reported a slight change in ADLs, in that he no longer participated in his favourite hobby of playing golf, but attributed that to increased motor difficulty rather than any cognitive change. He felt that his problems with concentration had developed over the last 12 months, and had not been present when he received his PD diagnosis. He reported a longstanding problem with his digestion, mainly taking the form of constipation, and difficulty in attaining good-quality sleep, although he did not report anything corresponding to REM sleep disorder.

BF had graduated from university and had a career in the civil service before retiring after being diagnosed with PD. He remained active in his retirement, playing golf until one year ago, and attending a local photographic society. He felt his motor problems had worsened considerably since his diagnosis, although he experienced some benefit from medication.

BF scored 85/100 on the ACE-III during his screening assessment and was referred for further cognitive testing. He received a fairly extensive battery, containing at least two tests of each aspect of cognitive function. His scores were reduced on both tests of processing speed (although this could be attributed at least partly to motor slowing), on one test of working memory/attention, and one test of executive function. These tests were greater than 1.5 standard deviations lower than expected on the basis of his estimated premorbid ability. Given these results, the pre-existing diagnosis of PD, and the absence of a decline in everyday function which could be attributed to a change in cognition, he was given a diagnosis of PD-MCI.

References

Aarsland, D., Ballard, C., Larsen, J. P., & McKeith, I. (2001). A comparative study of psychiatric symptoms in dementia with Lewy bodies and Parkinson's disease with and without dementia. *International Journal of Geriatric Psychiatry*, **16**(5), 528–36.

Aarsland, D., Zaccai, J., & Brayne, C. (2005). A systematic review of prevalence studies of dementia in Parkinson's disease. *Movement Disorders: Official Journal of the Movement Disorder Society*, **20**(10), 1255–63.

Albert, M. S., DeKosky, S. T., Dickson, D., et al. (2011). The diagnosis of mild cognitive impairment due to Alzheimer's disease: Recommendations from the National Institute on Aging–Alzheimer's Association workgroups on diagnostic guidelines for Alzheimer's disease. *Alzheimer's & Dementia*, 7(3), 270–9.

Aldridge, G. M., Birnschein, A., Denburg, N. L., & Narayanan, N. S. (2018). Parkinson's disease dementia and dementia with Lewy bodies have similar neuropsychological profiles. *Frontiers in Neurology*, 9, 323049.

Anang, J. B., Gagnon, J. F., Bertrand, J. A., et al. (2014). Predictors of dementia in Parkinson disease: A prospective cohort study. *Neurology*, 83(14), 1253–60.

Armstrong, M. J., Litvan, I., Lang, A. E., et al. (2013). Criteria for the diagnosis of corticobasal degeneration. *Neurology*, 80(5), 496–503.

Benito-León, J., Bermejo-Pareja, F., Rodríguez, J., et al. (2003). Prevalence of PD and other types of parkinsonism in three elderly populations of central Spain. *Movement Disorders*, 18(3), 267–74.

Ben-Shlomo, Y., Wenning, G. K., Tison, F., & Quinn, N. P. (1997). Survival of patients with pathologically proven multiple system atrophy: A meta-analysis. *Neurology*, 48(2), 384–93.

Berg, D., Postuma, R. B., Adler, C. H., et al. (2015). MDS research criteria for prodromal Parkinson's disease. *Movement Disorders*, 30(12), 1600–11.

Bonelli, S. B., Ransmayr, G., Steffelbauer, M., et al. (2004). L-dopa responsiveness in dementia with Lewy bodies, Parkinson disease with and without dementia. *Neurology*, **63**(2), 376–8.

Braak, H., Del Tredici, K., Rüb, U., et al. (2003). Staging of brain pathology related to sporadic Parkinson's disease. *Neurobiology of Aging*, **24**(2), 197–211.

Brockmann, K., Srulijes, K., Pflederer, S., et al. (2015). GBA-associated Parkinson's disease: Reduced survival and more rapid progression in a prospective longitudinal study. *Movement Disorders*, 30(3), 407–11.

Cammisuli, D. M., Cammisuli, S. M., Fusi, J., Franzoni, F., & Pruneti, C. (2019). Parkinson's disease–mild cognitive impairment (PD-MCI): A useful summary of update knowledge. *Frontiers in Aging Neuroscience*, 11, 303.

Chan, P. C., Lee, H. H., Hong, C. T., Hu, C. J., & Wu, D. (2018). REM sleep behavior disorder (RBD) in dementia with Lewy bodies (DLB). *Behavioural Neurology*, **2018**, ID 9421098. https://doi.org/10.1155/2018/9421098.

Cools, R. (2006). Dopaminergic modulation of cognitive function-implications for L-DOPA treatment in Parkinson's disease. *Neuroscience & Biobehavioral Reviews*, **30**(1), 1–23.

Cummings, J. L. (1988). Intellectual impairment in Parkinson's disease: Clinical, pathologic, and biochemical correlates. *Topics in Geriatrics*, 1(1), 24–36.

de Lau, L. M., Schipper, C. M. A., Hofman, A., Koudstaal, P. J., & Breteler, M. M. (2005). Prognosis of Parkinson disease: Risk of dementia and mortality: The Rotterdam Study. *Archives of Neurology*, 62(8), 1265–9.

Dickson, D. W., Bergeron, C., Chin, S. S., et al. (2002). Office of Rare Diseases neuropathologic criteria for corticobasal degeneration. *Journal of Neuropathology & Experimental Neurology*, 61(11), 935–46.

Downes, J. J., Priestley, N. M., Doran, M., et al. (1998). Intellectual, mnemonic, and frontal functions in dementia with Lewy bodies: A comparison with early and advanced Parkinson's disease. *Behavioural Neurology*, 11(3), 173–83.

Dubois, B., & Pillon, B. (1997). Cognitive deficits in Parkinson's disease. *Journal of Neurology*, **244**, 2–8.

Emre, M., Aarsland, D., Brown, R., et al. (2007). Clinical diagnostic criteria for dementia associated with Parkinson's disease. *Movement disorders: Official Journal of the Movement Disorder Society*, **22**(12), 1689–707.

Filoteo, J. V., Salmon, D. P., Schiehser, D. M., et al. (2009). Verbal learning and memory in patients with dementia with Lewy bodies or Parkinson's disease with dementia. *Journal of Clinical and Experimental Neuropsychology*, **31**(7), 823–34.

Friedman, J. H. (2017). Misperceptions and Parkinson's disease. *Journal of the Neurological Sciences*, **374**, 42–6.

Gaig, C., Valldeoriola, F., Gelpi, E., et al. (2011). Rapidly progressive diffuse Lewy body disease. *Movement Disorders*, **26**(7), 1316–23.

Gallagher, C. (2019). Imaging in Parkinson's disease: Imaging studies can differentiate Parkinson's from other causes of Parkinsonism. *Practical Neurology*, **35**, 29–31.

Gerstenecker, A. (2017). The neuropsychology (broadly conceived) of multiple system atrophy, progressive supranuclear palsy, and corticobasal degeneration. *Archives of Clinical Neuropsychology*, **32**(7), 861–75.

Gibb, W. R., & Lees, A. (1988). The relevance of the Lewy body to the pathogenesis of idiopathic Parkinson's disease. *Journal of Neurology, Neurosurgery & Psychiatry*, **51**(6), 745–52.

Gomperts, S. N. (2016). Lewy body dementias: Dementia with Lewy bodies and Parkinson disease dementia. *Continuum: Lifelong Learning in Neurology*, **22**(2), 435.

Gnanalingham, K. K., Byrne, E. J., Thornton, A., Sambrook, M. A., & Bannister, P. (1997). Motor and cognitive function in Lewy body dementia: Comparison with Alzheimer's and Parkinson's diseases. *Journal of Neurology, Neurosurgery & Psychiatry*, **62**(3), 243–52.

Gurd, J. M., Herzberg, L., Joachim, C., et al. (2000). Dementia with Lewy bodies: A pure case. *Brain and Cognition*, **44**(3), 307–23.

Hely, M. A., Morris, J. G., Reid, W. G., & Trafficante, R. (2005). Sydney multicenter study of Parkinson's disease: Non-L-dopa-responsive problems dominate at 15 years. *Movement Disorders: Official Journal of the Movement Disorder Society*, **20**(2), 190–9.

Hobson, P., & Meara, J. (2004). Risk and incidence of dementia in a cohort of older subjects with Parkinson's disease in the United Kingdom. *Movement Disorders*, **19**(9), 1043–9.

Hogan, D. B., Fiest, K. M., Roberts, J. I., et al. (2016). The prevalence and incidence of dementia with Lewy bodies: A systematic review. *Canadian Journal of Neurological Sciences*, **43**(S1), S83–S95.

Höglinger, G. U., Respondek, G., Stamelou, M., et al. (2017). Clinical diagnosis of progressive supranuclear palsy: The movement disorder society criteria. *Movement Disorders*, **32**(6), 853–64.

Hu, M. T. (2020). REM sleep behavior disorder (RBD). *Neurobiology of Disease*, **143**, 104996.

Hughes, T. A., Ross, H. F., Musa, S., et al. (2000). A 10-year study of the incidence of and factors predicting dementia in Parkinson's disease. *Neurology*, **54**(8), 1596–603.

Iansek, R., & Dandoudis, M. (2019). Parkinson's disease. In D. Hocking, J. Bradshaw & J. Fielding (Eds.), *Degenerative Disorders of the Brain* (pp. 65–87). Oxford: Routledge.

Jankovic, J., & Aguilar, L. G. (2008). Current approaches to the treatment of Parkinson's disease. *Neuropsychiatric Disease and Treatment*, **4**(4), 743.

Janvin, C. C., Larsen, J. P., Aarsland, D., & Hugdahl, K. (2006). Subtypes of mild cognitive impairment in Parkinson's disease: Progression to dementia. *Movement Disorders: Official Journal of the Movement Disorder Society*, **21**(9), 1343–9.

Jellinger, K. A. (2018). Dementia with Lewy bodies and Parkinson's disease-dementia: current concepts and controversies. *Journal of Neural Transmission*, **125**(4), 615–50.

Kao, A. W., Racine, C. A., Quitania, L. C., et al. (2009). Cognitive and neuropsychiatric profile of the synucleinopathies: Parkinson's disease, dementia with Lewy bodies and multiple system atrophy. *Alzheimer Disease and Associated Disorders*, **23**(4), 365.

Kim, W. S., Kågedal, K., & Halliday, G. M. (2014). Alpha-synuclein biology in Lewy body diseases. *Alzheimer's Research & Therapy*, **6**(5), 1–9.

Koga, S., Parks, A., Kasanuki, K., et al. (2017). Cognitive impairment in progressive supranuclear palsy is associated with tau burden. *Movement Disorders*, **32**(12), 1772–9.

Kouri, N., Murray, M. E., Hassan, A., et al. (2011). Neuropathological features of corticobasal degeneration presenting as corticobasal syndrome or Richardson syndrome. *Brain*, **134**(11), 3264–75.

Lagarde, J., Valabrègue, R., Corvol, J.-C., et al. (2013). Are frontal cognitive and atrophy patterns different in PSP and bvFTD? A comparative neuropsychological and VBM study. *PLoS ONE*, **8**(11), e80353. https://doi.org/10.1371/journal .pone.0080353.

Litvan, I., Aarsland, D., Adler, C. H., et al. (2011). MDS Task Force on mild cognitive impairment in Parkinson's disease: Critical review of PD-MCI. *Movement Disorders*, **26**(10), 1814–24.

Litvan, I., Agid, Y., Calne, D., et al. (1996). Clinical research criteria for the diagnosis of progressive supranuclear palsy (Steele-Richardson-Olszewski syndrome): Report of the NINDS-SPSP international workshop. *Neurology*, **47**(1), 1–9.

Litvan, I., Goldman, J. G., Tröster, A. I., et al. (2012). Diagnostic criteria for mild cognitive impairment in Parkinson's disease: Movement Disorder Society Task Force guidelines. *Movement Disorders*, **27**(3), 349–56.

McKeith, I. G., Boeve, B. F., Dickson, D. W., et al. (2017). Diagnosis and management of dementia with Lewy bodies: Fourth consensus report of the DLB Consortium. *Neurology*, **89**(1), 88–100.

McKeith, I., Mintzer, J., Aarsland, D., et al. (2004). International Psychogeriatric Association expert meeting on DLB: Dementia with Lewy bodies. *Lancet Neurology*, **3**(1), 19–28.

Morens, D. M., Davis, J. W., Grandinetti, A., et al. (1996). Epidemiologic observations on Parkinson's disease: Incidence and mortality in a prospective study of middle-aged men. *Neurology*, **46**(4), 1044–50.

Moretti, D. V. (2019). Available and future treatments for atypical parkinsonism. A systematic review. *CNS Neuroscience & Therapeutics*, **25**(2), 159–74.

Mosimann, U. P., Mather, G., Wesnes, K. A., et al. (2004). Visual perception in Parkinson disease dementia and dementia with Lewy bodies. *Neurology*, **63**(11), 2091–6.

Mouton, A., Blanc, F., Gros, A., et al. (2018). Sex ratio in dementia with Lewy bodies balanced between Alzheimer's disease and Parkinson's disease dementia: A cross-sectional study. *Alzheimer's Research & Therapy*, **10**(1), 1–10.

Nalls, M. A., Duran, R., Lopez, G., et al. (2013). A multicenter study of glucocerebrosidase mutations in dementia with Lewy bodies. *JAMA Neurology*, **70**(6), 727–35.

Nath, U., Ben-Shlomo, Y., Thomson, R. G., Lees, A. J., & Burn, D. J. (2003). Clinical features and natural history of progressive supranuclear palsy: A clinical cohort study. *Neurology*, **60**(6), 910–16.

Nelson, H. E. (1982). *National Adult Reading Test (NART): Test manual.* Windsor: NFER-Nelson.

Nomura, T., Inoue, Y., Mitani, H., et al. (2003). Visual hallucinations as REM sleep behavior disorders in patients with Parkinson's disease. *Movement Disorders*, **18**(7), 812–17.

Ossenkoppele, R., Jansen, W. J., Rabinovici, G. D., et al. (2015). Prevalence of amyloid PET positivity in dementia syndromes: A meta-analysis. *JAMA*, **313**(19), 1939–50.

Parkinson's UK (2018). The incidence and prevalence of Parkinson's in the UK Results from the Clinical Practice Research Datalink Summary report. www.parkinsons.org.uk/sit es/default/files/2018-01/CS2960%20Incidenc e%20and%20prevalence%20report%20brand ing%20summary%20report.pdf.

Phongpreecha, T., Cholerton, B., Mata, I. F., et al. (2020). Multivariate prediction of dementia in Parkinson's disease. *NPJ Parkinson's Disease*, **6**(1), 1–10.

Pillon, B., Deweer, B., Agid, Y., & Dubois, B. (1993). Explicit memory in Alzheimer's, Huntington's, and Parkinson's diseases. *Archives of Neurology*, **50**(4), 374–79.

Pirozzolo, F. J., Hansch, E. C., Mortimer, J. A., Webster, D. D., & Kuskowski, M. A. (1982). Dementia in Parkinson disease: A neuropsychological analysis. *Brain and Cognition*, **1**(1), 71–83.

Pagano, G., Niccolini, F., & Politis, M. (2016). Imaging in Parkinson's disease. *Clinical Medicine*, **16**(4), 371.

Postuma, R. B., Berg, D., Stern, M., et al. (2015). MDS clinical diagnostic criteria for Parkinson's disease. *Movement disorders*, **30**(12), 1591–601.

Postuma, R. B., Berg, D., Adler, C. H., et al. (2016). The new definition and diagnostic criteria of Parkinson's disease. *The Lancet Neurology*, **15**(6), 546–8.

Potashkin, J. A., Santiago, J. A., Ravina, B. M., Watts, A., & Leontovich, A. A. (2012). Biosignatures for Parkinson's disease and atypical Parkinsonian disorders patients. *PLoS ONE* 7(8), e43595. https://doi.org/10.1371/journal.pone.0043595.

Palavra, N. C., Naismith, S. L., & Lewis, S. J. (2013). Mild cognitive impairment in Parkinson's disease: A review of current concepts. *Neurology Research International, 2013*. 576091. https://doi.org/10.1155/2013/576091.

Ruffmann, C., Calboli, F. C., Bravi, I., et al. (2016). Cortical Lewy bodies and Aβ burden are associated with prevalence and timing of dementia in Lewy body diseases. *Neuropathology and Applied Neurobiology*, **42**(5), 436–50.

Sadiq, D., Whitfield, T., Lee, L., et al. (2017). Prodromal dementia with Lewy bodies and prodromal Alzheimer's disease: A comparison of the cognitive and clinical profiles. *Journal of Alzheimer's Disease*, **58**(2), 463–70.

Saeed, U., Lang, A. E., & Masellis, M. (2020). Neuroimaging advances in Parkinson's disease and atypical Parkinsonian syndromes. *Frontiers in Neurology*, 1189.

Salthouse, O., Bradshaw, J., & Saling, M. (2019). Dementia with Lewy bodies. In D. Hocking, J. Bradshaw, & J. Fielding (Eds.), *Degenerative Disorders of the Brain* (pp. 186–98). Oxford: Routledge.

Savica, R., Grossardt, B. R., Bower, J. H., et al. (2013). Incidence of dementia with Lewy bodies and Parkinson disease dementia. *JAMA Neurology*, **70**(11), 1396–402.

Schoenberg, M., & Duff, K. (2011). Dementias and mild cognitive impairment in adults. In M. Schoenberg & J. Scott (Eds), *The Little Black Book of Neuropsychology* (pp. 357–404). London; Springer.

Sekiya, H., Koga, S., Otsuka, Y., et al. (2022). Clinical and pathological characteristics of later onset multiple system atrophy. *Journal of Neurology*, **269**, 4310–21.

Schadlu, A. P., Schadlu, R., & Shepherd III, J. B. (2009). Charles Bonnet syndrome: A review. *Current Opinion in Ophthalmology*, **20**(3), 219–22.

Stanford, P. M., Halliday, G. M., Brooks, W. S., et al. (2000). Progressive supranuclear palsy pathology caused by a novel silent mutation in exon 10 of the tau gene: Expansion of the disease phenotype caused by tau gene mutations. *Brain*, **123**(5), 880–93.

Stankovic, I., Krismer, F., Jesic, A., et al. (2014). Cognitive impairment in multiple system atrophy: A position statement by the Neuropsychology Task Force of the MDS Multiple System Atrophy (MODIMSA) study group. *Movement Disorders*, **29**(7), 857–67.

Takao, M., Ghetti, B., Yoshida, H., et al. (2004). Early-onset dementia with Lewy bodies. *Brain Pathology*, **14**(2), 137–47.

Van Rooden, S. M., Heiser, W. J., Kok, J. N., et al. (2010). The identification of Parkinson's disease subtypes using cluster analysis: a systematic review. *Movement Disorders*, **25**(8), 969–78.

Vasconcellos, L. F. R., & Pereira, J. S. (2015). Parkinson's disease dementia: Diagnostic criteria and risk factor review. *Journal of Clinical and Experimental Neuropsychology*, **37**(9), 988–93.

Vergouw, L. J., van Steenoven, I., van de Berg, W. D., et al. (2017). An update on the genetics of dementia with Lewy bodies. *Parkinsonism & Related Disorders*, 43, 1–8.

Walker, L., Stefanis, L., & Attems, J. (2019). Clinical and neuropathological differences between Parkinson's disease, Parkinson's disease dementia and dementia with Lewy bodies – Current issues and future directions. *Journal of Neurochemistry*, **150**(5), 467–74.

Wenning, G. K., Litvan, I., Jankovic, J., et al. (1998). Natural history and survival of 14 patients with corticobasal degeneration confirmed at postmortem examination. *Journal of Neurology, Neurosurgery, and Psychiatry*, 4, 184–9.

Wenning, G. K., Stankovic, I., Vignatelli, L., et al. (2022). The movement disorder society criteria for the diagnosis of multiple system atrophy. *Movement Disorders*, **37**(6), 1131–48.

Williams, M. M., Xiong, C., Morris, J. C., & Galvin, J. E. (2006). Survival and mortality differences between dementia with Lewy bodies vs Alzheimer disease. *Neurology*, **67**(11), 1935–41.

Williams-Gray, C. H., Evans, J. R., Goris, A., et al. (2009). The distinct cognitive syndromes of Parkinson's disease: 5 year follow-up of the CamPaIGN cohort. *Brain*, **132**(11), 2958–69.

Williams-Gray, C. H., Mason, S. L., Evans, J. R., et al. (2013). The CamPaIGN study of Parkinson's disease: 10-year outlook in an incident population-based cohort. *Journal of Neurology, Neurosurgery & Psychiatry*, **84**(11), 1258–64.

Wu, T., Kansaku, K., & Hallett, M. (2004). How self-initiated memorized movements become automatic: A functional MRI study. *Journal of Neurophysiology*, **91**(4), 1690–8.

Yip, A. G., Brayne, C., & Matthews, F. E. (2006). Risk factors for incident dementia in England and Wales: The Medical Research Council Cognitive Function and Ageing Study. A population-based nested case-control study. *Age and Ageing*, **35**(2), 154–60.

Zaccai, J., McCracken, C., & Brayne, C. (2005). A systematic review of prevalence and incidence studies of dementia with Lewy bodies. *Age and Ageing*, **34**(6), 561–6.

Frontotemporal Dementia

Frontotemporal dementias are a collection of disorders which are associated with degeneration of the frontal and temporal lobes. They are usually young onset, and are associated with abnormal tau proteins. The three most common forms are a fontal variant, commonly referred to as behavioural variant (bvFTD) and two language-based variants known as primary progressive aphasias (PPA). The more anterior presentation is agrammatical/non-fluent (nfvPPA), and the more posterior presentation is known as semantic dementia (SD). A third form, logopenic PPA, is more commonly associated with Alzheimer-type pathology. Right hemisphere temporal lobe variants are also found, although their clinical presentation tends to be more diverse. These sometimes present clinically as a behavioural variant or with deficits associated with right hemisphere lesions such as prosopagnosia (impaired face recognition), which makes diagnosis more challenging (Josephs et al., 2009). Right hemisphere patients with predominantly temporal lobe atrophy who present with bvFTD tend to have more frontal atrophy than those with SvPPA (left hemisphere). Most cases of svPPA present with bilateral temporal lobe atrophy, whereas nfvPPA shows a stronger pattern of asymmetrical atrophy towards the left (Rogalski et al., 2011). In addition, FDT can occur within the context of a movement disorder. Up to 15% of FTD patients will go on to develop motor neuron disease (MND), and up to 30% of MND patients will develop FTD (Lomen-Hoerth, 2011). Cortical-basal degeneration and progressive supranuclear palsy, which are atypical Parkinsonian syndromes, also present with FTD (Josephs et al., 2006).

Prevalence and Incidence

The behavioural variant is the most common form of FTD, accounting for roughly 60% of cases (Onyike & Diehl-Schmidt, 2013). Ratnavelli et al. (2002) reported a prevalence of 15 per 100,000 in the population aged 45–64, which was the same as for Alzheimer's disease in that age range. Other studies have reported Alzheimer's disease to be the more common presentation for young-onset dementia (Knopman & Roberts, 2011). Average age of onset for FTD was 52.8 years. Although they found a strong male predominance, this has not been reported in all studies; 25% of cases have been noted to occur after the age of 65 (Onyike & Schmid, 2013). Survival time post diagnosis varies considerably according to the different subtype, with SD having a median survival of 12 years (Nunneman et al., 2011), whereas bvFTD and nfvPPA have a median survival time of 9 years (Robertson et al., 2005). MND-FTD is associated with a more rapid progression and shorter median survival time of 3 years (Hodges et al., 2003).

Toxic Agent

FTDs are usually considered to be tauopathies, although they are associated with a number of different protein types, including tau (FTLD-tau) and TAR-DNA binding protein 43 (TDP-43; FTLD-TDP) and fused-in-sarcoma (FUS; FTLD-FUS) (MacKenzie & Neumann, 2016; Neumann et al., 2009). The disorder was originally referred to as Pick's disease and was associated with characteristic cell types which became referred to as Pick's bodies; this terminology was abandoned as it was found that only 20% of cases had this type of pathology (Brun, 1993). The identification of these different proteins is based solely on post-mortem studies at the moment. It is currently not possible to identify a protein-based subtype while the person is alive.

Genetics and Other Risk Factors

FTD is familial in 30–50% of cases (Bird et al., 2003), with up to 40% of cases being autosomal dominant (Goldman et al., 2005), and at least five gene locations having been identified for causal mutations (Onyike & Diel-Schmid, 2013). FTD-MND is reported to be the most inheritable form, and svPPA the least (Goldman et al., 2005). In cases of sporadic FTD, the APOE4 gene has not been shown to have as strong a relationship as with some other forms of dementia. Rosso et al. (2002) reported that 6% of their FTD patients had this gene, as opposed to 2.6% of non-dementia patients. It was more common in the temporal lobe variant (9.7%) than the frontal variant (4.5%).

A number of studies have looked for non-genetic risk factors for the development of FTD. A history of traumatic brain injury was a risk factor for developing FTD, whereas the relevance of vascular risk was roughly the same as for other forms of dementia (Kalkonde et al., 2012). No association was found between smoking and FTD, although there was some association with obesity (Eid et al., 2019). Anxiety has been associated with development of FTD, but not Alzheimer's, whereas depression has been associated with development of Alzheimer's but not FTD (Rasmussen et al., 2018). Around 10.2–11.6% of patients with bvFTD have a history of bipolar disorder (Roman Meller et al., 2021).

bvFTD

This is the most common form of FTD and is initially characterised by changes in behaviour, personality, and executive function. The types of behavioural changes are those associated with damage to the frontal lobes, and are often observed in other forms of pathology such as traumatic brain injury. Alexander first described five circuits linking the basal ganglia, thalamus, and frontal lobes (Alexander, 1994; Alexander & Crutcher, 1990), two of which are concerned with motor control and three of which are related to cognition and behaviour. The dorsolateral prefrontal circuit supports the cognitive aspects of executive function, and most neuropsychological tests assessing executive function depend upon the integrity of this area (Lichter & Cummings, 2001). The orbitofrontal circuit is involved with social cognition (Cicerone & Tanenbaum, 1997) and damage to this circuit is associated with disinhibition. The anterior cingulate circuit is concerned with mechanisms of motivation, and damage to this circuit is associated with apathy/lack of initiation (Bonelli & Cummings, 2007). It is possible to have selective damage to these pathways, so somebody presenting with disinhibition/socially inappropriate behaviour may still score reasonably well on a set of executive assessments. It is also possible that these pathways may be affected in different combinations.

The marked personality changes have sometimes led to patients initially being misdiagnosed as having a psychiatric illness, particularly if there is little evidence of frontal atrophy seen on a scan (Lanata & Miller, 2016). A study of 252 consecutive referrals to a dementia clinic found that 52.2% of patients with FTD had initially been diagnosed with a psychiatric disorder and were more likely to have been initially diagnosed with schizophrenia or bipolar disorder than were other neurodegenerative disorders (Wooley et al., 2011). Although hallucinations and delusions are not typical FTD presentations, psychotic symptoms are reported in roughly 10% of patients (Swartz et al., 1997). The question of whether there might be a common genetic underpinning for both FTD and schizophrenia was considered by Schoder et al. (2010) by looking at first-degree relatives of 100 individuals with familial FTD and 100 with familial AD. They reported a significantly higher rate of schizophrenia in the relatives of those with FTD.

Interestingly, there are reports of a non-progressive variant of bvFTD, which is difficult to distinguish clinically from progressive bvFTD. These patients have normal structural imaging and are less impaired on activities of daily living, tests of executive function, and tests of social cognition (Kipps, Hodges, & Horberger, 2010). They are unlikely to have a degenerative disorder, although it is uncertain exactly what their aetiology might be.

Pattern of Atrophy

In the early stages of the disease, structural imaging is often unremarkable even though symptoms may be present. When volume loss becomes detectable, it is usually first seen in the orbitofrontal cortex (Perry et al., 2006), which is consistent with the early presentation of the disorder. Broe et al. (2003) put forward a staging system based upon post-mortem examination of 24 patients. This consisted of

1. mild atrophy in the orbital cortex, superior medial frontal cortices, and the hippocampus
2. progression to anterior frontal cortex, basal ganglia and temporal cortices
3. spread to all remaining tissue in these areas
4. marked atrophy in all areas

Progression of atrophy over the course of a year was found to be greater in bvFTD and svPPA than in AD (Krueger et al., 2010).

Diagnostic Criteria

Following on from previous criteria by Neary et al. (1998), the International Behavioural Variant FTD Criteria Consortium (FTDC) developed revised guidelines for the diagnosis of bvFTD (Rascovsky et al., 2011).

The first requirement is for evidence of a neurodegenerative disorder, as shown by progressive deterioration of behaviour and/or cognition by observation or history.

Following this, there are a range of cognitive and/or behavioural criteria, at least three of which are required within the first three years for a diagnosis of *possible* bvFTD.

- Behavioural disinhibition
- Apathy or inertia
- Loss of sympathy or empathy

- Perseverative, stereotypical, or compulsive behaviour

Two more criteria may present slightly later:

- Hyperorality and changes to diet
- Executive deficits, in the context of relatively well-preserved memory and visual-spatial function.

Probable bvFTD requires the addition of evidence of functional decline either by carer report or rating scale, and CT/MRI/PET evidence consistent with bvFTD.

Exclusion criteria are patterns of deficits better accounted for by other non-degenerative neurological disorders, or psychiatric disorder. Hallmarks of AD are also an exclusion criterion.

Guidelines for pathologically confirmed FTD require histological evidence or the presence of a known pathogenic mutation.

Cognitive Assessment

A neuropsychological assessment is likely to be vital in this diagnosis; however, this is not always straightforward as measurable cognitive deficits may not be apparent in the early stages due to the disease presenting in the orbital cortex, whereas most neuropsychology tests of executive function measure dorsolateral prefrontal function. Most research in this area has tended to concentrate less on whether cognitive testing can detect evidence of a decline in executive function, and more on distinguishing FTD from AD. The standard finding has been that FTD patients show more impairment on tests of executive function, with less impairment on tests of memory, whereas patients with AD show the opposite pattern (Walker et al., 2005). FTD patients show relative preservation of visuospatial/ constructional abilities (Rascovsky et al., 2011). There is also evidence that there are different cognitive profiles associated with different genes, which is again related to the relative severity of executive and memory deficits (Poos et al., 2020).

Although work has been carried out using extensive neuropsychological assessments, there is always a call for briefer tools which take up less clinical time. Mathuranath et al. (2000) looked at using the ACE-II for the purpose of discriminating FTD from AD, developing the VLOM ratio based upon combining some subtests into indices which consist of ([verbal fluency + language] / [orientation + memory]). A score of <2.2 is indictive of FTD, and a score of >3.2 is indicative of AD. It should be noted that this research was conducted using ACE-R rather than ACE-II. Although the difference between the two instruments was the replacement of items from the then newly copyrighted MMSE (Folstein, Folstein, & McHugh 1975) with equivalent items, the study has not been repeated with the ACE-III.

The concepts of social cognition and theory of mind have existed in psychology for some decades, influencing research on animal cognition (Premack & Woodruff, 1978), autism (Baron-Cohen, 1997), and language development (Astington & Jenkins, 1999), but have been slow to influence neuropsychological practice. This may be partly due to the availability of tests of these concepts normed to the same extent as standardised tests of cognition. Although not designed for use in dementia settings, several tests are being considered in disorders such as FTD where these abilities become impaired relatively early. Recognition of facial emotion has been studied quite extensively in degenerative disorders, including FTD. Keane et al. (2002) reported that that patients with FTD were impaired in recognition of facial expression, but not facial identity. Bora, Vellakunis, and Waterfang (2016) performed a meta-analysis comparing patients with FTD to AD and controls. They were significantly impaired in recognition of negative emotions when compared to controls, and more impaired with recognition of all emotions other than happiness when compared to AD. The Ekman faces are often used for this purpose (Ekman & Friesen, 1976). The Awareness of Social Inference Test (TASIT) (McDonald et al., 2003) is a test involving the inference of emotion from watching videos, which is used in clinical practice. Kipps et al. (2009) compared bvFTD, AD, and controls, reporting that FTD patients (with imaging evidence) were impaired on recognition of negative emotions and sarcasm; patients with AD and controls did not experience difficulty with either of these.

Kertesz et al. (2003) compared FTD and AD patients on a battery of neuropsychological tests, and a frontal behavioural inventory. AD patients had lower memory scores, whereas FTD patients had lower language scores. Although they were able to correctly classify 78% of patients on the basis of cognitive test scores, they were able to correctly classify 98% on the basis of the behavioural inventory. A number of different inventories have been developed for assessing behavioural change, which are predominantly carer-based as loss of insight (anamnesis) is a common finding in FTD. Examples of inventories specifically aimed at frontal lobe changes are the Frontal Behavioural Inventory (Kertesz, Davidson, & Fox, 1997) and the Frontal Systems Behavioural Scale (Duff et al., 2010).

Primary Progressive Aphasia

PPA are a group of initially language-based disorders, which have been described for many years (Pick, 1892) but only categorised relatively recently (Mesulam, 2001; Gorno-Tempini et al., 2011). There are three identifiable types of PPA, currently referred to as non-fluent variant (nfvPPA), semantic variant (svPPA), and logopenic variant (lvPPA). Spinelli et al. (2017) looked at the frequency of different proteinopathies in a sample of 69 patients with sporadic PPA and reported each variant to be associated with a specific clinical, imaging, and pathological variant. All svPPA patients showed primary FTLD pathology, 88% of lvPPA patients showed primary FTLD pathology, and all lvPPA had primary AD pathology. Secondary pathologies were also evident in some patients.

How Do PPAs Relate to Classical (Stroke-Based) Models of Aphasia?

For those who find it useful to relate these presentations to classical models, there is fortunately some overlap, although the correspondence may not be exact.

- nfvPPA aligns most closely with Broca's aphasia
- svPPA aligns most closely with transcortical sensory aphasia (i.e. speech repetition preserved)
- lvPPA aligns most closely with Wernicke's or conduction aphasia (i.e. speech repetition impaired) (Marshall et al., 2018)

Prevalence, Genetics, and Disease Progression

Although PPA is thought to comprise up to 40% of cases of FTD, it is still a comparatively rare disorder, with an estimated prevalence of 3 cases per 100,000 (Coyle-Gilchrist et al., 2016). Ramos et al. (2019) carried out screening for the main causative and risk variant genes in a sample of 403 PPA patients. Causative genes were found in only 14/403 cases, most commonly in nfvPPA (5.6%). Only 2 cases were seen in svPPA and 1 in logopenic PPA; 28.3% of the cohort carried at least one APOE4 allele, with the biggest concentration being in the lvPPA patients (36%). The conclusion was that both causative and risk-associated genes are rarely involved in PPA. Although not linked to a specific gene, there have been reports of higher incidence of learning disabilities in relatives of patients with PPA. Rogalski et al. (2014) reported that in a case series of 66 patients followed up post-mortem, 50% had either a personal or family history of language-based learning disability (including dyslexia).

The diagnosis of different forms of PPA is based primarily on their initial presentation, although there is evidence that as they develop, they follow quite distinct patterns. Ulugut et al. (2022) followed up 64 biomarker-confirmed cases of PPA over a period of up to 6 years, observing some consistency in the way the different subtypes evolved. nfvPPA typically progressed towards mutism, and developed motor deficits, with roughly half meeting the diagnostic criteria for PSP, CBD, or MND after a period of 5 years. lvPPA developed wider language and cognitive problems, with 83% coming to meet the diagnostic criteria for AD. svPPA retained the primary difficulty in semantic processing but were more likely to develop behavioural problems, with 58% eventually meeting the criteria for bvFTD. Although PPAs initially present with language disorders, the deficits do not remain exclusively language-based as the disease progresses.

Clinical Diagnosis of PPA

At present, there is a two-stage diagnostic process analogous to that for diagnosing dementia. Stage 1 involves determining whether the person meets the criteria for PPA. Once PPA is established, stage 2 involves identifying the subtype. It is important for things to proceed in that order, as the deficits seen in PPA are often also found with other degenerative disorders (e.g. AD). The important requirement for PPA is that the language disorder is the initial presenting feature and retains a greater relative degree of severity than other features which may develop as the disease progresses.

Mesulam (2001) outlined the original criteria, of which there were seven:

1. Gradual onset of problems with word-finding, object naming, or word comprehension
2. No impairment in activities of daily living which is not attributable to the language deficit for at least two years post-onset
3. No evidence of premorbid language difficulties (other than dyslexia)
4. No evidence of apathy/disinhibition, problems with episodic memory, non-verbal memory, visuospatial processing, or sensory-motor dysfunction in the first two years post onset
5. Dyspraxia and acalculia may be present in the first two years
6. After the first two years, other aspects of cognition may be affected but the language deficit remains primary and progresses at a greater rate than other aspects of impairment
7. Absence of other causes such as stroke/tumour evidenced by imaging.

Diagnosing the Subtype

The original classification system required a relatively straightforward distinction between fluent and non-fluent aphasia. However, a third category called logopenic PPA was introduced by Gorno-Tempini et al. (2004), which is widely accepted and has good clinical validity as it is usually found to be associated with AD-type pathology rather than tau.

Whilst it can be relatively straightforward to distinguish nfvPPA from the fluent svPPA, the difference in clinical presentation between lpvPPA and svPPA is often not clear (Rascovsky & Grossman, 2013). There is also a subset of patients who do not seem to map on well to these categories and are hence referred to as 'unclassifiable' (Utianski et al., 2019), although their imaging data suggest that the affected brain regions are no different to the classifiable presentations.

Semantic Variant

The defining feature of svPPA is that it is a disorder of semantic memory, whereby the meanings of words and objects are lost, alongside general and personal knowledge. svPPA was the earliest identified and most extensively studied form of PPA. First described by Pick (1892), interest accelerated following three cases studied by Warrington (1975), who demonstrated agnosia (inability to recognise objects), anomia (problems with word-finding), and impaired verbal comprehension. A series of five patients were described by Mesulum (1982), which gave rise to the term 'primary progressive aphasia'. Snowden, Goulding, and Neary (1989) coined the phrase 'semantic dementia' to describe this group of patients, which was followed by diagnostic criteria in 1992 (Hodges et al., 1992).

Current diagnostic criteria (Gorno-Tempini et al., 2011) list the following requirements. All criteria list the necessity of clinical diagnosis and imaging-supported diagnosis. A pathologically confirmed diagnosis also requires histopathological evidence of a degenerative pathogen or the presence of a known pathogenic mutation.

Whilst there are papers emphasising a more qualitative means of diagnosis (e.g. Marshall et al., 2018), the clinical criteria are best evaluated with the use of formal tests.

1) Clinical diagnosis:

   The core features, both of which are required, are impaired confrontation naming and impaired single word comprehension.

   Three of the following are also required:

   - Impaired object knowledge, especially for low frequency items
   - Surface dyslexia or dysgraphia
   - Spared speech repetition
   - Spared speech production. Speech must be grammatical and free flowing, although need not make any sense
2) Imaging-supported diagnosis:

   - Clinical diagnosis of svPPA plus prominent anterior temporal lobe atrophy, or anterior temporal lobe hypoperfusion or hypometabolism evidenced by PET or SPECT.

Evidencing the Clinical Diagnosis

A large number of language tests have been developed over the years, very few of which are standardised to an extent which is comparable to tests of cognition used by neuropsychologists. Some suggestions are made here for assessment tools to use, although interpretation of results will be a mixture of quantitative and qualitative information.

Confrontation naming. This is typically assessed with a picture-naming task, of which there are many available with varying degrees of standardisation. The Boston Naming test (Kaplan, Goodglass, & Weintraub, 1983) is probably the best known and most widely used (Rabin, Barr, & Burton, 2005).

Single word comprehension. This can be assessed formally by picture–word matching. Marshall et al. (2018) suggest asking the patient to describe an object or pick it out from an array,

Impaired object knowledge (especially low frequency words). Semantic association tests such as the Pyramids and Palm Trees (Howard & Patterson, 1992) can be used to assess object knowledge. This test presents three pictures: one on top and two underneath. The participant must identify which of the two underneath is semantically related to the one at the top (e.g. a pyramid at the top, and a palm tree and a pine tree underneath).

Surface dyslexia. Normal reading proceeds on the basis of spelling–sound correspondences and word meanings. If the meanings are no longer available, it may still proceed based on spelling–sound correspondences (i.e. sounding words out). However, this will only work for words with regular spellings, whereas English has many irregular spellings for which this will not work. The presence of surface dyslexia can therefore be assessed by asking the patient to read a list of words with regular and irregular spellings. A higher error rate should be apparent for irregular words.

Spared speech repetition. This can be tested by requesting the patient to repeat single words and sentences.

Spared speech production. This can be assessed via spontaneous conversation, or asking the patient to describe something such as a picture (e.g. The Cookie Thief test from the Boston Diagnostic Aphasia Examination; Goodglass, Kaplan, & Barresi, 2001).

nfvPPA

The non-fluent variant maps relatively closely onto the classical aphasia syndrome of Broca's aphasia, the core features of which are slow, laboured speech production and agrammatism consisting of short, simple phrases often without function words. Whilst comprehension of single words is generally intact, comprehension of syntax is often impaired. Word-finding difficulties are very different to those seen in svPPA, where the person is unable to retrieve the required word. With nfvPPA, the person can retrieve the word but is unable to articulate it.

Diagnostic Criteria

Gorno-Tempini et al. (2011) list the following requirements.

1. Clinical diagnosis:

   The core features are agrammatism in speech production and laboured, effortful speech. Only one of these is required.

   At least two of the following:

- Impaired comprehension of syntactically complex sentences
- Preserved object knowledge
- Preserved single word comprehension

2. Imaging-supported diagnosis requires a clinical diagnosis of nfvPPA, with the addition of predominant left posterior fronto-insular atrophy on MRI *or* predominant left posterior fronto-insular hypoperfusion or hypometabolism on SPECT or PET.

Evidencing the Clinical Diagnosis for nfvPPA

Agrammatical speech production and/or laboured speech. These may be apparent in spontaneous speech, or when describing a picture. As there is a difficulty generating the motor programmes to articulate speech, there will often be a word length effect, with difficulty in articulation increasing along with word length.

Impaired comprehension of syntactically complex sentences. This can be assessed using tests such as sentence–picture matching, as found in the Psycholinguistic Assessment of Language Processing in Aphasia (PALPA; Kay, Coltheart, & Lesser, 1992). This involves matching a sentence to one of three pictures, with the word order being crucial to selecting the correct one (e.g. the girl chased the chicken).

Preserved object knowledge. This can be assessed with a semantic association task.

Preserved single word comprehension. This can be assessed via picture–word matching.

lvPPA

This is the most recent addition to the subtypes of PPA, and is often considered to be the most challenging to diagnose as there can be some degree of overlap with the other two forms (Marshall et al., 2018). As it is usually an atypical variant of AD, there may be other cognitive deficits present at a relatively early stage which could inform diagnosis, although none are as yet part of the diagnostic criteria (Savage et al., 2013).

Diagnostic Criteria

1. Clinical diagnosis:
   The core features, both of which are required, are impaired single word retrieval in spontaneous speech and naming, and impaired repetition of single words and sentences.

At least three of the following must be present:

- phonological errors in spontaneous speech and naming
- spared single word comprehension and object knowledge
- spared motor speech
- absence of agrammatism
2. Imaging-supported diagnosis requires additional predominant posterior left perisylvian or parietal atrophy on MRI, or predominant posterior left perisylvian or parietal hypoperfusion or hypometabolism on SPECT or PET.

Evidencing Clinical Diagnosis of LvPPA

Impaired single word retrieval in spontaneous speech and naming. This can be assessed either in spontaneous speech or via a picture-naming test

Table 8.1 Clinical features of PPA subtypes

Clinical feature	nfvPPA	svPPA	lvPPA
Agrammatism	Yes	No	No
Motor speech/articulation problems	Yes	No	No
Single word comprehension problems	No	Yes	No
Impaired comprehension of syntax	Yes	No	No
Problems with object recognition/knowledge	No	Yes	No
Surface dyslexia	No	Yes	No
Phonological errors in spontaneous speech	No	No	Yes
Impaired single word retrieval in spontaneous speech	No	Yes	Yes
Problems repeating speech	Yes (with multi-syllabic and phonologically similar words)	No	Yes

Impaired repetition of single words and sentences. This can be assessed formally using tests from batteries such as the PALPA (Kay, Coltheart, & Lesser, 1992).

Phonological errors in spontaneous speech and naming. Phonological errors refer to an error in speech production based around the sound of the word. This can be assessed via spontaneous speech or picture naming.

Spared single word comprehension and object knowledge. This can be assessed by picture–word matching or semantic association.

Spared motor speech. This can be assessed with spontaneous speech or describing a picture

Absence of agrammatism. No evidence of articulation problems or agrammatism should be present in spontaneous speech or describing a picture.

A summary of clinical features is displayed in Table 8.1.

In terms of the reliability of clinical signs, there is evidence that some tend to be more reliable than others. There has also been some investigation of cognitive abilities not currently included in the diagnostic criteria, such as digit span. Leyton et al. (2014b) compared verbal repetition across the different subtypes, finding that all groups showed some difficulty, with lvPPA demonstrating the most severe effect and svPPA experiencing the least difficulty and only with sentences. svPPA did not differ significantly from controls for digit span, whereas lvPPA and nfvPPA were impaired. In a second study, Leyton et al. (2014a) reported that the most reliable features to discriminate between 'non-semantic' variants of PPA were phonological errors in lvPPA and motor speech/agrammatism in nfvPPA.

Key Points

- FTD refers to a number of degenerative disorders which mainly affect the frontal and temporal lobes. Onset in most cases is before the age of 65.
- FTDs are associated with a number of different forms of tauopathy, and a number of cases have been associated with specific genes. Roughly 40% follow an autosomal dominant pattern.
- FTD quite frequently presents within the context of a movement disorder, such motor neurone disease, corticobasal degeneration, or progressive supranuclear palsy.
- bvFTD accounts for roughly 60% of cases, and is associated with atrophy of the frontal-striatal systems. It usually presents with behavioural changes, such as disinhibition or apathy. Scores on neuropsychological tests of executive function can often be unaffected in the early stages.
- There are three forms of PPA, two of which are related to tauopathies (svPPA and nfvPPA) and are forms of FTD. The more recently identified lvPPA is more consistently associated with Alzheimer pathology.
- Whilst nfvPPA can be quite distinctively characterised by agrammatic speech and difficulties with articulation, and svPPA is characterised by difficulties in single word comprehension, lvPPA can be more difficult to identify. It has been suggested that the presence of phonological errors in speech is the most reliable distinguishing feature.

Appendix I Case Studies

Case Study: MH

MH was a 63-year-old female with a long-term history of bipolar disorder, who was admitted to a psychiatric ward with lithium toxicity. She lived alone following the death of her husband four months earlier, after which she had displayed a number of difficulties including not managing her medication. Concerns were raised following a routine visit by a community psychiatric nurse. She had previously run a local shop with her husband, but following his death had not felt able to continue and closed the business. Her next of kin was her son, who worked shifts and was not available to give a detailed history or complete any questionnaires regarding behavioural/cognitive change. Her community psychiatric nurse had known her for a number of years and felt that she had been heavily supported by her husband and had not coped well following his death. She felt there had always been example of slightly unusual behaviour related to her bipolar disorder.

During her stay on the ward, some unusual behaviours were noticed. At mealtimes, she tended to continually put food into her mouth before swallowing the previous mouthful, which had led to several episodes of choking that required urgent intervention by staff. She chain-smoked unless her access to cigarettes was monitored by staff, and when smoking a cigarette she took very deep inhalations, which meant that each one was finished very quickly. She was independent with self-care, other than requiring the occasional prompt. A CT scan was requested, which reported 'no abnormality found', and she was subsequently referred for a neuropsychology assessment.

MH had little formal education, leaving school at 15 without formal qualifications, and had married at 16 (with parental consent). She and her husband ran their shop until his death four months before her hospital admission. Her neuropsychology assessment was difficult to interpret as her estimated premorbid ability fell at the cusp of Borderline/Low Average, and none of her cognitive tests gave results significantly lower than this.

The initial hypothesis was that MH had functioned well because of the extent of support she received from her husband and had probably managed the less demanding duties around the shop. The factor which made the difference to her level of function was the removal of this lifelong support. This was discussed with her son, who was unhappy with this conclusion, and provided more information at this point.

MH had in fact held quite a high level of responsibility in the shop and took joint responsibility for managing and ordering stock. Her son reported that there had been some changes in her behaviour prior to the death of her husband and gave examples of possible disinhibition. There was also some family history of dementia, although the type was not specified. An MRI scan was requested at this stage, which reported widening of sulci within the frontal lobes. The diagnosis was therefore revised to bvFTD.

Case Study: PS

PS was a 66-year-old female who presented to her GP with a two-year history of memory complaints and word-finding difficulties. There had been a gradual onset, with the word-finding problems being described as more severe than the memory problems. She scored below cut-off on the screening instrument used in clinic, but it was noted that she performed particularly badly on the language-based subtests, which resulted in her attaining a score that would normally be considered indicative of dementia. During the clinical interview, word-finding problems and circumlocutions were evident in spontaneous speech. An MRI scan described mild bilateral temporal lobe atrophy, more pronounced in the left hemisphere.

PS had completed a degree, then trained as a primary school teacher. Her final post before retirement was as a deputy head teacher. She was married with two adult children, both of whom lived locally. She was generally independent with activities of daily living, although she no longer enjoyed socialising due to difficulties holding a conversation.

She was referred for a neuropsychology and language assessment. Given that she presented with language problems, it was not considered appropriate to use a reading-based test to estimate premorbid ability. On the basis of her demographic variables, her premorbid ability was estimated to fall within the Average to High Average range. She completed the WAIS-IV, scoring well on perceptual reasoning tests, but scored a little bit lower on the other indices. Her digit span was notably low. She completed a verbal memory and a visual memory test, scoring lower than expected for verbal memory and within the expected range for visual memory. There was a reduced output for verbal fluency, but no difference between letter and category fluency. Performance on a non-verbal reasoning test did not indicate any impairment.

Language tests revealed difficulties in picture naming, but also an imperfect score for picture–word matching and semantic association, suggesting some semantic difficulties. There was no evidence of agrammatic speech production or difficulties with articulation, which ruled out nfvPPA. Speech repetition was unimpaired for single words, but the occasional error was observed when repeating sentences. There was no evidence of surface dyslexia. There was also no evidence of phonological errors in speech production.

Although not a perfect match, it was considered that the most likely diagnosis was svPPA.

References

Alexander, G. E. (1994). Basal ganglia-thalamocortical circuits: Their role in control of movements. *Journal of Clinical Neurophysiology: Official Publication of the American Electroencephalographic Society*, **11**(4), 420–31.

Alexander, G. E., & Crutcher, M. D. (1990). Functional architecture of basal ganglia circuits: Neural substrates of parallel processing. *Trends in Neurosciences*, **13**(7), 266–71.

Astington, J. W., & Jenkins, J. M. (1999). A longitudinal study of the relation between language and theory-of-mind development. *Developmental Psychology*, **35**(5), 1311.

Baron-Cohen, S. (1997). *Mindblindness: An Essay on Autism and Theory of Mind*. Cambridge, MA: MIT Press.

Bird, T., Knopman, D., VanSwieten, J., et al. (2003). Epidemiology and genetics of frontotemporal dementia/Pick's disease. *Annals of Neurology*, **54**, S29–S31.

Bonelli, R. M., & Cummings, J. L. (2007). Frontal-striatal circuitry and behaviour. *Dialogues in Clinical Neuroscience*, **9**(2), 141–51.

Bora, E., Velakoulis, D., & Walterfang, M. (2016). Meta-analysis of facial emotion recognition in behavioral variant frontotemporal dementia: Comparison with Alzheimer disease and healthy controls. *Journal of Geriatric Psychiatry and Neurology*, **29**(4), 205–11.

Broe, M., Hodges, J. R., Schofield, E., et al. (2003). Staging disease severity in pathologically confirmed cases of frontotemporal dementia. *Neurology*, **60**(6), 1005–11.

Brun, A. (1993). Frontal lobe degeneration of non-Alzheimer type revisited. *Dementia*, **4**, 126–31.

Cicerone, K. D., & Tanenbaum, L. N. (1997). Disturbance of social cognition after traumatic orbitofrontal brain injury. *Archives of Clinical Neuropsychology*, **12**(2), 173–88.

Coyle-Gilchrist, I. T., Dick, K. M., Patterson, K., et al. (2016). Prevalence, characteristics, and survival of frontotemporal lobar degeneration syndromes. *Neurology*, **86**(18), 1736–43.

Duff, K., Paulsen, J. S., Beglinger, L. J., et al. (2010). 'Frontal' behaviors before the diagnosis of Huntington's disease and their relationship to markers of disease progression: Evidence of early lack of awareness. *The Journal of Neuropsychiatry and Clinical Neurosciences*, **22**(2), 196–207.

Eid, H. R., Rosness, T. A., Bosnes, O., et al. (2019). Smoking and obesity as risk factors in frontotemporal dementia and Alzheimer's disease: The HUNT Study. *Dementia and Geriatric Cognitive Disorders Extra*, **9**(1), 1–10.

Ekman, P., & Friesen, W. V. (1976). *Pictures of Facial Affect*. Palo Alto: Consulting Psychologists Press.

Folstein, M. F., Folstein, S. E., & McHugh, P. R. (1975). 'Mini-mental state': A practical method for grading the cognitive state of patients for the clinician. *Journal of Psychiatric Research*, **12**(3), 189–98.

Goldman, J. S., Farmer, J. M., Wood, E. M., et al. (2005). Comparison of family histories in FTLD subtypes and related tauopathies. *Neurology*, **65**(11), 1817–19.

Goodglass, H., Kaplan, E., & Barresi, B. (2001). *Boston Diagnostic Aphasia Examination*. 3rd ᵉd. Baltimore: Lippincott, Williams & Wilkins.

Gorno-Tempini, M. L., Dronkers, N. F., Rankin, K. P., et al. (2004). Cognition and anatomy in three variants of primary progressive aphasia. *Annals of Neurology: Official Journal of the American Neurological Association and the Child Neurology Society*, **55**(3), 335–46.

Gorno-Tempini, M. L., Hillis, A. E., Weintraub, S., et al. (2011). Classification of primary progressive aphasia and its variants. *Neurology*, **76**(11), 1006–14.

Hodges, J. R., Davies, R., Xuereb, J., Kril, J., & Halliday, G. (2003). Survival in frontotemporal dementia. *Neurology*, **61**(3), 349–54.

Hodges, J. R., Patterson, K., Oxbury, S., & Funnell, E. (1992). Semantic dementia: progressive fluent aphasia with temporal lobe atrophy. *Brain*, **115**, 1783–806.

Howard, D., & Patterson, K. (1992). *The Pyramids and Palm Trees: A test of Semantic Access from Pictures and Words*. Bury St Edmunds: Thames Valley Test Company.

Josephs, K. A., Petersen, R. C., Knopman, D. S., et al. (2006). Clinicopathologic analysis of frontotemporal and corticobasal degenerations and PSP. *Neurology*, **66**(1), 41–8.

Josephs, K. A., Whitwell, J. L., Knopman, D. S., et al. (2009). Two distinct subtypes of right temporal variant frontotemporal dementia. *Neurology*, **73**(18), 1443–50.

Kalkonde, Y. V., Jawaid, A., Qureshi, S. U., et al. (2012). Medical and environmental risk factors associated with frontotemporal dementia: A case-control study in a veteran population. *Alzheimer's & Dementia*, **8**(3), 204–10.

Kaplan, E., Goodglass, H., & Weintraub, S. (1983). *Boston Naming Test*. Philadelphia: Lea & Febiger.

Kay, J., Coltheart, M., & Lesser, R. (1992). *PALPA: Psycholinguistic Assessments of Language Processing in Aphasia*. New York: Psychology Press.

Keane, J., Calder, A. J., Hodges, J. R., & Young, A. W. (2002). Face and emotion processing in frontal variant frontotemporal dementia. *Neuropsychologia*, **40**(6), 655–65.

Kertesz, A., Davidson, W, & Fox H. (1997). Frontal behavioral inventory: Diagnostic criteria for frontal lobe dementia. *Canadian Journal of Neurological Sciences*, **24**, 29–36.

Kipps, C. M., Hodges, J. R., & Hornberger, M. (2010). Nonprogressive behavioural frontotemporal dementia: Recent developments and clinical implications of the 'bvFTD phenocopy syndrome'. *Current Opinion in Neurology*, **23**(6), 628–32.

Kipps, C. M., Nestor, P. J., Acosta-Cabronero, J., Arnold, R., & Hodges, J. R. (2009). Understanding social dysfunction in the behavioural variant of frontotemporal dementia: The role of emotion and sarcasm processing. *Brain*, **132**(3), 592–603.

Knopman, D. S., & Roberts, R. O. (2011). Estimating the number of persons with frontotemporal lobar degeneration in the US population. *Journal of Molecular Neuroscience*, **45**, 330–5.

Krueger, C. E., Dean, D. L., Rosen, H. J., et al. (2010). Longitudinal rates of lobar atrophy in frontotemporal dementia, semantic dementia, and Alzheimer's disease. *Alzheimer Disease & Associated Disorders*, **24**(1), 43–8.

Lanata, S. C., & Miller, B. L. (2016). The behavioural variant frontotemporal dementia (bvFTD) syndrome in psychiatry. *Journal of Neurology, Neurosurgery & Psychiatry*, **87**(5), 501–11.

Leyton, C. E., Ballard, K. J., Piguet, O., & Hodges, J. R. (2014a). Phonologic errors as a clinical marker of the logopenic variant of PPA. *Neurology*, **82**(18), 1620–7.

Leyton, C. E., Savage, S., Irish, M., et al. (2014b). Verbal repetition in primary progressive aphasia and Alzheimer's disease. *Journal of Alzheimer's Disease*, **41**(2), 575–85.

Lichter, D. G., & Cummings, J. L. (2001). Introduction and overview. In D. G. Lichter, & J. L. Cummings (Eds.). *Frontal-Subcortical Circuits in Psychiatric and Neurological Disorders* (pp. 1–43). Guilford Press.

Lomen-Hoerth, C. (2011). Clinical phenomenology and neuroimaging correlates in ALS-FTD. *Journal of Molecular Neuroscience*, **45**(3), 656–62.

Mackenzie, I. R., & Neumann, M. (2016). Molecular neuropathology of frontotemporal dementia: insights into disease mechanisms from postmortem studies. *Journal of Neurochemistry*, **138**, 54–70.

Mackenzie, I. R., Neumann, M., Baborie, A., et al. (2011). A harmonized classification system for FTLD-TDP pathology. *Acta Neuropathologica*, **122**(1), 111–13.

Marshall, C. R., Hardy, C. J., Volkmer, A., et al. (2018). Primary progressive aphasia: A clinical approach. *Journal of Neurology*, **265**(6), 1474–90.

Mathuranath, P. S., Nestor, P. J., Berrios, G. E., Rakowicz, W., & Hodges, J. R. (2000). A brief cognitive test battery to differentiate Alzheimer's disease and frontotemporal dementia. *Neurology*, **55**(11), 1613–20.

McDonald, S., Flanagan, S., Rollins, J., & Kinch J. (2003). TASIT: A new clinical tool for assessing social perception after traumatic brain injury. *Journal of Head Injury Trauma Rehabilitation*, **18**, 219–38.

Mesulam, M. (1982). Slowly progressive aphasia without generalised dementia. *Annals of Neurology*, **11**, 592–98.

Mesulam, M. M. (2001). Primary progressive aphasia. *Annals of Neurology*, **49**(4), 425–32.

Neary, D., Snowden, J. S., Gustafson, L., et al. (1998). Frontotemporal lobar degeneration: A consensus on clinical diagnostic criteria. *Neurology*, **51**(6), 1546–54.

Neumann, M., Rademakers, R., Roeber, S., et al. (2009). A new subtype of frontotemporal lobar degeneration with FUS pathology. *Brain*, **132**(11), 2922–31.

Nunnemann, S., Last, D., Schuster, T., Förstl, H., Kurz, A., & Diehl-Schmid, J. (2011). Survival in a German population with frontotemporal lobar degeneration. *Neuroepidemiology*, **37** (3–4), 160–5.

Onyike, C. U., & Diehl-Schmid, J. (2013). The epidemiology of frontotemporal dementia. *International Review of Psychiatry*, **25**(2), 130–7.

Perry, R. J., Graham, A., Williams, G., et al. (2006). Patterns of frontal lobe atrophy in frontotemporal dementia: A volumetric MRI study. *Dementia and Geriatric Cognitive Disorders*, **22**(4), 278–87.

Pick A. (1892). Ueber die Beziehungen der senilen Hirnatrophie zur Aphasie. *Prager Med Wochenschr*, **17**, 165–7.

Poos, J. M., Jiskoot, L. C., Leijdesdorff, S. M. J., et al. (2020). Cognitive profiles discriminate between genetic variants of behavioral frontotemporal dementia. *Journal of Neurology*, **267**(6), 1603–12.

Premack, D., & Woodruff, G. (1978). Does the chimpanzee have a theory of mind? *Behavioral and Brain Sciences*, **1**(4), 515–26.

Rabin, L. A., Barr, W. B., & Burton, L. A. (2005). Assessment practices of clinical neuropsychologists in the United States and Canada: A survey of INS, NAN, and APA Division 40 members. *Archives of Clinical Neuropsychology*, **20**(1), 33–65.

Ramos, E. M., Dokuru, D. R., Van Berlo, V., et al. (2019). Genetic screen in a large series of patients with primary progressive aphasia. *Alzheimer's & Dementia*, **15**(4), 553–60.

Rascovsky, K., & Grossman, M. (2013). Clinical diagnostic criteria and classification controversies in frontotemporal lobar degeneration. *International Review of Psychiatry*, **25**(2), 145–58.

Rascovsky, K., Hodges, J. R., Knopman, D., et al. (2011). Sensitivity of revised diagnostic criteria for the behavioural variant of frontotemporal dementia. *Brain*, **134**(9), 2456–77.

Rasmussen, H., Rosness, T. A., Bosnes, O., et al. (2018). Anxiety and depression as risk factors in frontotemporal dementia and Alzheimer's disease: The HUNT study. *Dementia and Geriatric Cognitive Disorders Extra*, **8**(3), 414–25.

Ratnavalli, E., Brayne, C., Dawson, K., & Hodges, J. R. (2002). The prevalence of frontotemporal dementia. *Neurology*, **58**(11), 1615–21.

Roberson, E. D., Hesse, J. H., Rose, K. D., et al. (2005). Frontotemporal dementia progresses to death faster than Alzheimer disease. *Neurology*, **65**(5), 719–25.

Rogalski, E. J., Rademaker, A., Wieneke, C., et al. (2014). Association between the prevalence of learning disabilities and primary progressive aphasia. *JAMA Neurology*, **71** (12), 1576–7.

Rogalski, E., Cobia, D., Harrison, T. M., et al. (2011). Progression of language decline and cortical atrophy in subtypes of primary progressive aphasia. *Neurology*, **76**(21), 1804–10.

Roman Meller, M., Patel, S., Duarte, D., Kapczinski, F., & de Azevedo Cardoso, T. (2021). Bipolar disorder and frontotemporal dementia: A systematic review. *Acta Psychiatrica Scandinavica*, **144**(5), 433–47.

Rosso, S. M., Van Swieten, J. C., Roks, G., et al. (2002). Apolipoprotein E4 in the temporal variant of frontotemporal dementia. *Journal of Neurology, Neurosurgery & Psychiatry*, **72** (6), 820.

Savage, S., Hsieh, S., Leslie, F., et al. (2013). Distinguishing subtypes in primary progressive aphasia: application of the Sydney language battery. *Dementia and Geriatric Cognitive Disorders*, **35**(3–4), 208–18.

Schoder, D., Hannequin, D., Martinaud, O., et al. (2010). Morbid risk for schizophrenia in first-degree relatives of people with frontotemporal dementia. *The British Journal of Psychiatry*, **197**(1), 28–35.

Snowden, J. S., Goulding, P. J., & Neary, D. (1989). Semantic dementia: A form of circumscribed cerebral atrophy. *Behavioural Neurology*, **2**, 167–82.

Spinelli, E. G., Mandelli, M. L., Miller, Z. A., et al. (2017). Typical and atypical pathology in primary progressive aphasia variants. *Annals of Neurology*, **81**(3), 430–43.

Swartz, J. R., Miller, B. L., Lesser, I. M., & Darby, A. L. (1997). Frontotemporal dementia: Treatment response to serotonin selective reuptake inhibitors. *Journal of Clinical Psychiatry*, **58**(5), 212–17.

Ulugut, H., Stek, S., Wagemans, L. E., et al. (2022). The natural history of primary progressive aphasia: Beyond aphasia. *Journal of Nneurology*, **269**(3), 1375–85.

Utianski, R. L., Botha, H., Martin, P. R., et al. (2019). Clinical and neuroimaging characteristics of clinically unclassifiable primary progressive aphasia. *Brain and Language*, **197**, 104676.

Walker, A. J., Meares, S., Sachdev, P. S., & Brodaty, H. (2005). The differentiation of mild frontotemporal dementia from Alzheimer's disease and healthy aging by neuropsychological tests. *International Psychogeriatrics*, **17**(1), 57–68.

Warrington, E. K. (1975). Selective impairment of semantic memory. (1975) *Quarterly Journal of Experimental Psychology*, **27**, 635–57.

Woolley, J. D., Khan, B. K., Murthy, et al. (2011). The diagnostic challenge of psychiatric symptoms in neurodegenerative disease: rates of and risk factors for prior psychiatric diagnosis in patients with early neurodegenerative disease. *The Journal of Clinical Psychiatry*, **72**(2), 126–33.

Alcohol-Related Brain Damage

Alcohol-related brain damage (ARBD) has historically been referred to by various different names, including alcohol-related dementia and Korsakoff's dementia. The current DSM-V refers to it as Alcohol-induced Neurocognitive Disorder, which may be seen as implying it is a form of dementia (Major Neurocognitive Disorder being the term used by DSM-V instead of dementia). However, it is not a dementia as it is possible to remove the toxic agent (alcohol), following which there is no further progression and even an improvement in function in many cases. In this respect it is more correctly classified as form of acquired brain injury, although where ARBD should sit in terms of healthcare pathways can be an area for debate.

Prevalence of ARBD

Most studies have considered ARBD prevalence in the context of dementia. One of the most cited studies was by Smith and Kiloh (1981), who reported that 'alcohol-related dementia (ARD)' accounted for 10% of all cases of dementia. Ritchie and Villebrun (2008) reported that between 9% and 22% of patients with dementia have a history of heavy alcohol use, and 10–24% of chronic heavy alcohol users would meet the criteria for dementia. Prevalence figures for ARBD tend to indicate that the age of onset is younger than for true dementias, with most cases being in the young and middle-aged parts of the population (Sachdeva et al., 2016) (i.e. prevalence rates do not show an age-related increase as seen in the most common forms of dementia). Harvey et al. (2003) carried out an epidemiological study of an English cohort of young-onset dementia cases (aged less than 65) and reported that ARD accounted for 10% of cases. Draper et al. (2011) reported that ARD accounted for 23% of cases of young-onset dementia in an Australian population. Gilchrist and Morrison (2005) looked at a sample of 266 homeless people in Glasgow. They concluded that 82% had cognitive impairment and 21% had ARBD. Kril and Harper (2012) reported that around 15% of people with chronic alcoholism have neurological signs of Korsakoff's. Galvin et al. (2010) concluded that roughly 10% of long-term alcohol consumers had Wernicke–Korsakoff Syndrome (WKS) on the basis of post-mortem studies.

Acquired Brain Injury

In cases of acquired brain injury, two processes occur:

1. Brain cells die. This may be due to the direct results of the injury (e.g. a traumatic impact) or secondary effects of the brain injury (e.g. swelling, lack of blood supply, or accumulation of blood). Once brain cells have died, we have no means of bringing them

back to life. There is no evidence-based treatment for brain injury which involves regenerating areas of the brain which have died.

2. Other brain cells survive but are temporarily not functioning. Spontaneous recovery following a brain injury involves these areas regaining function.

The situation is slightly more complex than this as it is possible to develop long-term reorganisation of function, known as plasticity, and brain injury rehabilitation is able to focus on relearning skills using compensatory strategies. ARBD also fits into this pattern as there is often a combination of irreversible deficits due to cell death, and a reversible component arising from networks of cells with impaired function beginning to work again once the toxic agent has been removed.

Why Was ARBD Considered to Be a Dementia?

The simple answer to this is that its presentation is usually characterised by a severe anterograde amnesia (inability to retain new information), and deficits in executive function. In many ways this resembles Alzheimer's disease, and at one point the disorder was referred to as Korsakoff's dementia (as well as Korsakoff's psychosis). Over the course of time, one of the key pathological elements involved in the disorder was identified as an encephalopathy (a diffuse disease of the brain which impacts upon function/structure) arising from a deficiency of thiamine (vitamin B1). The evolution of our understanding of Wernicke–Korsakoff's syndrome is illustrated in Figure 9.1.

Why Is ARBD Better Characterised As a Form of Brain Injury?

One of the definitions of dementia is that it is progressive. An acquired brain injury (ABI) results from a process affecting the structure or function of the brain, but which does not progress. In fact, in most cases of ABI there is a degree of improvement, albeit rarely to the extent of reaching premorbid levels. Whilst ARBD can be progressive if the person continues to consume alcohol (the toxic agent), it has been claimed that abstaining from alcohol consumption can lead to a complete recovery of function within two years in cases who did not develop WKS (Stavro, Pelletier, & Potkin, 2013).

It could be argued that practically, as well as conceptually, it makes more sense to consider ARBD as a form of ABI as these patients tend to be younger and demonstrate a higher level of long-term rehabilitation potential that patents with dementia.

1881 – German psychiatrist Carl Wernicke describes the acute state of encephalopathy, characterised by eye movement disturbance, ataxia, and mental confusion. Cause unknown.

1887 – Russian Psychiatrist Sergei Korsakoff published the first of a series of papers describing the syndrome which would subsequently be termed Korsakoff's.

1901 – Karl Bonhoeffer links the these together, recognising Korsakoff's syndrome as the long-term consequence of Wernicke's encephalitis.

1912 – The concept of vitamins was first developed

1926 – Thiamine (vitamin B) identified and artificially synthesised in 1936

1952 – The role of thiamine identified in Wernicke's encephalopathy

1966 – Thiamine used in the treatment of Wernicke's encephalopathy

Figure 9.1 Time course of understanding the links between Wernicke's encephalopathy, Korsakoff's Syndrome, and Thiamine.

The Toxic Agents: Thiamine Deficiency and Alcohol-Related Neurotoxicity

There is evidence for two toxic processes at work in ARBD (Arts, Wallvoort, & Kessels, 2017):

1. Thiamine (vitamin B1) deficiency (TD) which can cause permanent irreversible damage, and
2. Ethanol-related neurotoxicity (EN), from which there can be significant improvement once consumption of alcohol has ceased.

Although it has been suggested that there is a continuum between EN and TD (Ryback, 1971; Butters & Brandt, 1985), there is strong evidence to suggest the two processes occur independently. The main difficulty with viewing these processes as part of the same continuum is that Korsakoff's syndrome arising from thiamine deficiency can occur in the absence of alcohol, due to conditions such as cancer, AIDS, gastrointestinal problems, and renal disorders (Scalzo et al., 2015), although most reported cases of WKS still occur in the context of heavy alcohol use.

If Wernicke's encephalopathy is correctly identified in the early stages and treated with intravenous thiamine, development of WKS can be prevented (Thomson, Guerrini, & Marshall, 2012). Interestingly, the required dose for treating alcoholic WKS is considerably higher than that required for non-alcoholic variants, which Thomson et al. attribute to other factors, such as impaired thiamine metabolism playing a role in alcoholic WKS. There is also a higher likelihood of developing the syndrome in times of sudden, unexpected alcohol withdrawal. Harper and Kril (1994) also suggested that alcoholic WKS may arise from multiple subclinical episodes of thiamine deficiency, rather than a single episode as seen in non-alcoholic WKS.

Arts et al. (2017) described five mechanisms whereby alcohol might facilitate the development of thiamine deficiency:

1. alcohol suppresses hunger
2. combustion of alcohol requires extra thiamine pyrophosphate
3. alcoholic gastroenteritis may impair absorption of thiamine
4. alcoholic liver disease impairs thiamine storage in the liver
5. alcohol may impair the utilisation of thiamine

EN is thought to have several possible mechanisms, but the main one is demyelination (Pereira, Andrade, & Valentao, 2015). The reversal of cognitive decline seen in many people with a sustained period of abstinence may be attributable to remyelination. If significant deficits remain following a period of sustained abstinence, it is likely that Wernicke's encephalopathy has occurred, even if it was not diagnosed at the time (Arts et al., 2017). For a brief revision of the role of myelin in the brain, see Chapter 3.

Neuroanatomy of WKS

There is a consensus that damage to the diencephalon is central to WKS. This is an area of the brain which includes the thalamus, the hypothalamus, the subthalamus, and the epithalamus. In two large autopsy studies, lesions to the mammillary bodies of the hypothalamus were seen in virtually all patients (Malamud & Skillicorn, 1956; Victor, Adams, & Collins, 1989). In post-mortem studies, the hippocampus has been reported to be smaller than that of controls, although the reduced volume seems to be due to a loss of white matter and was seen less in patients who had been abstinent at the time of death (Harding et al., 1997). Although several different brain areas have been implicated in WKS there has been some uncertainty whether damage to these additional areas is necessary to bring about the disorder. In their review of the literature, Kril and Harding (2012) concluded that damage to the anterior thalamus and the mamillary bodies of the hypothalamus is required, although WKS could also arise from damage to the interconnections between these and other areas. Whilst thiamine deficiency is considered to mainly affect these diencephalic regions (Jacobsen & Lishman, 1990; Fama, Pitel, & Sullivan, 2012), ethanol neurotoxicity is considered to have more effect on frontal lobe circuits (Fujiwara et al., 2008).

Cognitive Sequelae of ARBD

The most widely researched and reported cognitive sequelae of ARBD is anterograde amnesia: difficulty in creating new memories (Fame, Pitel, & Sullivan, 2012; Kopelman, 1995). Retrograde amnesia (the inability to recall memories from the period prior to the onset of the brain injury) is less severely affected, and displays a temporal gradient (Albert, Butters, & Levin, 1979; Seltzer & Benson, 1974). The deficit has been reported to be more severe for episodic memory than semantic memory (Kopelman, 1995; Verfaellie et al., 1992). Procedural learning, which usually involves the acquisition of a new skill, has been reported to be relatively well-preserved in Korsakoff's (Brooks & Baddeley, 1976; Talland, 1965).

Another hallmark of ARBD, particularly WKS, is confabulation, which is the tendency to create false memories (Borsutzky et al., 2008). Van Damme and d'Ydewalle (2010) looked at the nature of confabulations in a sample of patients and found the confabulations mainly occurred in response to questions about episodic memory and to questions where the patient did not know the answer. Confabulation in general is considered to arise when there are deficits in both memory and executive processes, with the severity of the executive deficit being the main predictor of whether confabulation will occur (Cunningham et al., 1997). Rensen et al. (2017) looked at this phenomenon in a group of 51 patients with Korsakoff's, finding that provoked confabulations (i.e. in response to a question) were associated with executive dysfunction and poorer memory performance: spontaneous confabulation was not related to performance tests of either executive function or memory.

Korsakoff's has long been associated with executive problems, although possibly not described as such because executive function has only been well-conceptualised in the last 40 years. Moerman-van den Brink et al. (2019) compared three aspects of executive function in 36 abstinent patients with Korsakoff's and 30 healthy controls. They found differences on set-shifting and updating, but not on tasks of inhibition. Other studies have reported Korsakoff's patients to be impaired on different aspects of executive function, including response inhibition, response generation, and planning (Brion et al., 2014; Van Oort & Kessels, 2009). Executive dysfunction has also been reported to play a contributory role in WKS memory difficulties as there are problems encoding information relating to spatial and temporal order (Postma et al., 2006). Korsakoff's patients typically have a lack of insight into their cognitive difficulties, which is also thought to be due to a deficit in executive function (Arts et al., 2017). Interestingly, non-alcoholic WKS patients reportedly retain better awareness of their cognitive deficits (Nikolakaros et al., 2016).

Diagnostic Criteria

Diagnosis of ARBD, or at least Korsakoff's, is complicated by the fact that there do not seem to be generally accepted diagnostic criteria (Arts et al., 2017; Gerridzen et al., 2017). ICD-11 and DSM-V differ slightly in their criteria. DSM-V considers *only* alcohol-related WKS and classifies it as 'alcohol-induced', which is potentially misleading (Arts et al., 2017). ICD-11 classifies alcoholic and non-alcoholic WKS separately, with the latter described as an organic mental disorder, and alcoholic WKS as a mental disorder due to substance abuse.

Wernicke's encephalopathy, the acute stage of the disorder, which can be thought of as a form of delirium, was originally diagnosed by the presence of (1) altered mental state and/or memory deficit, (2) nystagmus, ophthalmoplegia, or other disordered eye movements, and (3) ataxia/gait disturbance (Wernicke, 1881). However, only 16% of cases present with all three symptoms, and up to 20% of confirmed cases show none of these (Harper, Giles, & Finlay-Jones, 1986). Caine et al. (1997) proposed criteria requiring at least two of the following to be present: (1) dietary deficiencies, (2) oculomotor abnormalities, (3) cerebellar dysfunction, (4) confusion/disorientation or memory impairment. Wijnia (2022) suggested that immediate diagnosis of Wernicke's encephalopathy may be missed because of guidelines on delirium not including thiamine deficiency as a possible cause, and delirium of any cause is not diagnosed in up to 70% of cases.

The DSM-V diagnostic criteria for Substance/Medication-Induced Major or Mild Neurocognitive Disorder are as follows:

1. The criteria are met for major or mild neurocognitive disorder.
2. The neurocognitive impairments do not occur exclusively during the course of a delirium and persist beyond the usual duration of intoxication and acute withdrawal.
3. The involved substance or medication and duration and extent of use are capable of producing the neurocognitive impairment.
4. The temporal course of the neurocognitive deficits is consistent with the timing of substance or medication use and abstinence (e.g. the deficits remain stable or improve after a period of abstinence).
5. The neurocognitive disorder is not attributable to another medical condition or is not better explained by another mental disorder.

Whilst not proposing diagnostic criteria, Arts et al. (2017) suggested a definition to guide further development of such criteria:

1. WKS is an irreversible condition caused by thiamine deficiency following incomplete recovery from Wernicke's encephalopathy.
2. It occurs predominantly (but not exclusively) in the context of alcohol abuse and malnutrition.
3. It is characterised by an abnormal mental state, with episodic memory disproportionately affected, while the individual remains alert and responsive.
4. Additional features include executive dysfunction, flattened affect, apathy, lack of insight, and confabulation. These may be absent in milder forms and non-alcoholic cases.

Key differences between ARBD and a degenerative disorder such as Alzheimer's disease are presented in Table 9.1. It should be borne in mind that it is possible to have comorbidity, particularly in older patients, and if there is progression in the face of sustained abstinence there is likely to be a second process such as Alzheimer's disease operating.

Table 9.1 Key differences between Wernicke–Korsakoff syndrome and Dementia of the Alzheimer type

Wernicke–Korsakoff syndrome (alcohol-related)	Dementia of the Alzheimer type (DAT)
Typical age of onset between 40 and 60	Typical age of onset over 65, and incidence increases with age
Occurs in the context of chronic alcohol use	Can occur in the context of chronic alcohol use, but <u>not</u> in the majority of cases
Sudden onset	Gradual onset developing over months or years
Presents with memory and executive problems. Confabulation is a hallmark	Initial presentation of difficulty encoding new information. Executive problems and confabulations may occur as the disease progresses, but are not an early feature
Imaging shows lesions concentrated around the thalamus	Imaging shows atrophy in concentrated the medial temporal lobe
With continued abstinence, does not get worse and may show improvement	Cognitive deterioration progresses over time

When to Carry Out a Neuropsychological Assessment

Although an assessment of cognitive function may be essential in the diagnosis of ABRD, the timing of the assessment is crucial to obtaining a valid result. In general, a comprehensive neuropsychological assessment should only be conducted if the patient is cognitively stable. In the case of WKS, this means assessment should be avoided during the encephalopathy stage of the illness, as this is a temporary state of delirium. Wijnia et al. (2016) recommended that this can be done after six weeks of abstinence, unless there are ongoing signs of delirium, which should be resolved before progressing.

In cases without a clear episode of encephalopathy, the key question is whether the individual is still drinking and how much. From the perspective of a neuropsychologist, the person should be abstinent for a period of at least six weeks. From the perspective of an addiction specialist, this may be considered a completely unrealistic requirement for the majority of cases. As 14 units of alcohol per week is frequently cited as a safe upper limit, a prolonged period with consumption below this level may be an acceptable compromise. If this is not possible, a comprehensive assessment is not advised, and a brief cognitive screen would be recommended instead.

Key Points

- ARBD is an umbrella term which includes irreversible conditions such as WK, and potentially reversible conditions caused by ethanol neurotoxicity (which causes demyelination).
- Wernicke's encephalopathy is caused by thiamine deficiency, which can respond well to treatment in the early stages. Korsakoff's syndrome is the long-term, chronic condition when the recovery from Wernicke's encephalopathy is incomplete.

- Whilst this most commonly occurs in the context of chronic alcoholism, non-alcoholic forms can arise as a result of thiamine deficiency in other contexts (e.g. eating disorders, cancer).
- The improvement seen following a period of abstaining from alcohol probably reflects remyelination due to the removal of ethanol neurotoxicity.
- ARBD is not a true form of dementia as it does not progress if the person continues to abstain.
- The hallmark of Korsakoff's is a severe anterograde amnesia. Other features (such as executive problems, apathy, a lack of insight, and confabulation) are not always seen.
- Neuroanatomically, the main area of damage is the thalamus and inter-related circuits.
- Comprehensive neuropsychological assessments are not recommended for individuals who continue to consume high levels of alcohol. In these cases, a brief cognitive screen would be more appropriate.

Appendix J Case Study

Case Study: MM

MM was a 52-year-old male who was found by the police wandering the streets in the early hours of the morning in a confused state. Despite being mid-winter, MM was not wearing warm clothing, and was disoriented to time and place. Given his apparent state of confusion, MM was taken to the nearest general hospital. Access to his medical notes revealed he had been known to addictions services for a number of years; however, a blood test did not reveal the presence of alcohol. The Addenbrooke's Cognitive Examination (ACE-III) was administered, on which he achieved a total score of 56, which is considerably below the recommended cut-off of 88/100 for clinical practice. Given MM's known history of alcohol use, he was placed on a course of intravenous thiamine and referred for an MRI scan.

History

As MM was well-known to services, it was possible to obtain a reasonably detailed history despite MM not being able to contribute much himself. He had left school at 16, without formal qualifications, and worked as a builder until his mid-thirties, when he incurred a moderate traumatic brain injury from an industrial accident. He did not return to work following this incident, although it was unclear whether this was a direct result of the accident as his alcohol intake also increased significantly during this period. He was first seen by addictions services, which is an opt-in service, approximately ten years after his accident. Although they identified a high level of vulnerability, MM did not wish to engage in any intervention-related work.

Presentation on Admission to Hospital

MM was disoriented to time and place and was unable to given any information about his activities over the last year. He was also not able to give any information regarding next of kin, and alternated between stating this was his ex-wife and his brother (it was believed he had in fact had no contact with either for a number of years). He was able to give his address.

His MRI scan described the following: 'There is hyperintensity around the third ventricle which extends to the mamillary bodies. This is in keeping with Wernicke's encephalopathy. Generalised involutional changes are most pronounced in the frontal lobes. Gliosis in the right frontal lobe is noted, which is due to previous damage.'

MM was treated with high doses of thiamine for several days, and then with an ongoing maintenance dose. After six weeks, only limited improvement was noted and he was referred for a neuropsychological assessment.

Further Assessment

Given MM's low score on the ACE-III, a relatively brief neuropsychological assessment was considered most appropriate. MM's premorbid ability was estimated to be towards the lower end of the Average range. His scores indicated decline in immediate and delayed memory, and attention. His scores on two tests of executive function also indicated a decline.

MM did not show evidence of confabulation, but demonstrated a pronounced lack of insight, stating frequently that there was nothing wrong with his memory. He also showed signs of possible apathy, as he appeared content to sit in the chair by his bed all day watching any programme on the ward television. Ward staff reported he was continent, and would get up whenever he needed the toilet, although he always needed some assistance with how to find it.

On the basis of his known long-term history of alcohol use, the report from his MRI scan indicating Wernicke's encephalopathy, his severe memory impairment, lack of insight, and apathy, he was diagnosed with WKS.

References

Albert, M. S., Butters, N., & Levin, J. (1979). Temporal gradients in the retrograde amnesia of patients with alcoholic Korsakoff's disease. *Archives of Neurology*, 36(4), 211–16.

Arts, N., Walvoort, S., & Kessels, R. (2017). Korsakoff's syndrome: A critical review. *Neuropsychiatric Disease and Treatment*, 13, 2875–90.

Bonhoeffer, K. (1901). *Die Akuten Geisteskrankheiten Der Gewohnheitstrinker.* Jena: Fischer.

Borsutzky, S., Fujiwara, E., Brand, M., & Markowitsch, H. J. (2008). Confabulations in alcoholic Korsakoff patients. *Neuropsychologia*, 46(13), 3133–43.

Brion, M., Pitel, A. L., Beaunieux, H., & Maurage, P. (2014). Revisiting the continuum hypothesis: Toward an in-depth exploration of executive functions in Korsakoff syndrome. *Frontiers of Human Neuroscience*, 8, 1–7.

Brooks, D. N., & Baddeley, A. D. (1976). What can amnesic patients learn? *Neuropsychologia*, 14, 111–22.

Butters, N., & Brandt, J. (1985). The continuity hypothesis: The relationship of long-term alcoholism to the Wernicke–Korsakoff syndrome. *Recent Developments in Alcoholism*, 3, 207–26.

Caine, D., Halliday, G. M., Kril, J. J., & Harper, C. G. (1997). Operational criteria for the classification of chronic alcoholics: Identification of Wernicke's encephalopathy. *Journal of Neurology, Neurosurgery and Psychiatry*, 62(1), 51–60.

Cunningham, J. M., Pliskin, N. H., Cassisi, J. E., Tsang, B., & Rao, S. M. (1997) Relationship between confabulation and measures of memory and executive function. *Journal of Clinical and Experimental Neuropsychology*, 19(6), 867–77.

Draper, B., Karmel, R., Gibson, D., Peut, A., & Anderson, P. (2011). Alcohol-related cognitive impairment in New South Wales hospital patients aged 50 years and over. *The Australian and New Zealand Journal of Psychiatry*, **45**(11), 985–92.

Fama, R., Pitel, A. L. & Sullivan, E. V. (2012). Anterograde episodic memory in Korsakoff syndrome. *Neuropsychological Review*, **22**(2), 93–104.

Fujiwara, E., Brand, M., Borsutzky, S., Steingass, H.-P., & Markowitsch, H. J. (2008). Cognitive performance of detoxified alcoholic Korsakoff syndrome patients remains stable over two years. *Journal of Clinical and Experimental Neuropsychology*, **30**, 576–87.

Galvin, R., Brathen, G., Ivashynka, A., et al. (2010). EFNS guidelines for diagnosis, therapy and prevention of Wernicke encephalopathy. *European Journal of Neurology*, **17**(12), 1408–18.

Gerridzen, I. J., Moerman-van den Brink, W. G., Depla, M. F., et al. (2017). Prevalence and severity of behavioural symptoms in patients with Korsakoff syndrome and other alcohol-related cognitive disorders: A systematic review. *International Journal of Geriatric Psychiatry*, **32**(3), 256–73.

Gilchrist, G., & Morrison, G. S. (2005). Prevalence of alcohol related brain damage among homeless hostel dwellers in Glasgow, *European Journal of Public Health*, **15**(6), 587–8.

Harding, A. J., Wong, A., Svoboda, M., Kril, J. J., & Halliday, G. M. (1997). Chronic alcohol consumption does not cause hippocampal neuron loss in humans. *Hippocampus*, **7**, 78–87.

Harper, C., & Kril, J. (1994). An introduction to alcohol-induced brain damage and its causes. *Alcohol and Alcoholism. Supplement*, **2**, 237–43.

Harper, C. G., Giles, M., & Finlay-Jones, R. (1986). Clinical signs in the Wernicke–Korsakoff complex: A retrospective analysis of 131 cases diagnosed at necropsy. *Journal of Neurology, Neurosurgery, & Psychiatry*, **49**, 341–5.

Harvey, R. J., Skelton-Robinson, M., & Rossor, M. N. (2003). The prevalence and causes of dementia in people under the age of 65 years. *Journal of Neurology, Neurosurgery, and Psychiatry*, **74**(9), 1206–9.

Jacobson, R. R., & Lishman, W. A. (1990). Cortical and diencephalic lesions in Korsakoff's syndrome: a clinical and scan study. *Psychological Medicine*, **20**, 63.

Kopelman, M. D. (1995). The Korsakoff syndrome. *British Journal of Psychiatry*, **166** (2), 154–73.

Korsakoff, S. S. (1887). Ob alkogol'nom paraliche [Disturbance of psychic function in alcoholic paralysis and its relation to the disturbance of the psychic sphere in multiple neuritis of nonalcoholic origin]. *Vestn Psikhiatrii*, **4**(2), 1–102.

Kril, J. J., & Harper, C. G. (2012). Neuroanatomy and neuropathology associated with Korsakoff's syndrome. *Neuropsychological Review*, **22**(2), 72–80.

Malamud, N., & Skillicorn, S. A. (1956). Relationship between the Wernicke and the Korsakoff syndrome. *Archives of Neurology and Psychiatry*, **76**, 585–96.

Moerman-Van Den Brink, W. G., Van Aken, L., Verschuur, E. M. L., et al. (2019). Executive dysfunction in patients with Korsakoff's syndrome: A theory-driven approach. *Alcohol and Alcoholism*, **54**(1), 23–9.

Nikolakaros, G., Ilonen, T., Kurki, T., et al. (2016). Non-alcoholic Korsakoff syndrome in psychiatric patients with a history of undiagnosed Wernicke's encephalopathy. *Journal of the Neurological Sciences*, **370**, 296–302.

Periera, R. B., Andrade, P. B., & Valentao, P. (2015). A comprehensive view of the neurotoxicity of the neurotoxicity mechanisms of cocaine and ethanol. *Neurotoxicity Research*, **28**, 253–67.

Postma, A., Van Asselen, M., Keuper, O., Wester, A., & Kessels, R. (2006). Spatial and temporal order memory in Korsakoff patients. *Journal of the International Neuropsychological Society*, **12**(3), 327–36.

Rensen, Y. C., Oosterman, J. M., Walvoort, S. J., Eling, P. A., & Kessels, R. P. (2017). Intrusions and provoked and spontaneous confabulations on memory tests in Korsakoff's syndrome. *Journal of Clinical and Experimental Neuropsychology*, **39**(2), 101–11.

Ritchie, K., & Villebrun, D. (2008). Epidemiology of alcohol-related dementia. *Handbook of Clinical Neurology*, **89**, 845–50.

Ryback, R. S. (1971). The continuum and specificity of the effects of alcohol on memory. A review. *Quarterly Journal for Studies on Alcohol*, **32**(4), 995–1016.

Sachdeva, A., Chandra, M., Choudhary, M., Dayal, P., & Anand, K. S. (2016). Alcohol-related dementia and neurocognitive impairment: A review study. *International Journal of High Risk Behaviors & Addiction*, **5**(3), e27976.

Scalzo, S. J., Bowden, S. C., Ambrose, M. L., Whelan, G., & Cook, M. J. (2015). Wernicke–Korsakoff syndrome not related to alcohol use: A systematic review. *Journal of Neurology, Neurosurgery and Psychiatry*, **86**(12), 1362–8.

Seltzer, B., & Benson, D. F. (1974). The temporal pattern of retrograde amnesia in Korsakoff's disease. *Neurology*, **26**(6), 527–30.

Smith, J. S., & Kiloh, L. G. (1981). The investigation of dementia: Results in 200 consecutive admissions. *Lancet*, **1**(8224), 824–7.

Stavro, K., Pelletier, J., & Potvin, S. (2013). Widespread and sustained cognitive deficits in alcoholism: A meta-analysis. *Addiction Biology*, **18**(2), 203–13.

Talland, G. A. (1965). *Deranged memory: A psychonomic study of the amnesic syndrome*. New York: Academic.

Thomson, A. D., Guerrini, I., & Marshall, E. J. (2012). The evolution and treatment of Korsakoff's syndrome: Out of sight, out of mind? *Neuropsychological Review*, **22**, 81–92.

Van Damme, I., & d'Ydewalle, G. (2010). Confabulation versus experimentally induced false memories in Korsakoff patients. *Journal of Neuropsychology*, **4**(2), 211–30.

Van Oort, R., & Kessels, R. P. C. (2009). Executive dysfunction in Korsakoff's syndome: time to revise the DSM criteria for alcohol-induced persisting amnestic disorder? *International Journal of Psychiatry in Clinical Practice*, **13**(1), 78–81.

Verfaellie, M., Milberg, W. P., Cermak, L. S., & Letourneau, L. L. (1992). Priming of spatial configurations in alcoholic Korsakoff's amnesia. *Brain and Cognition*, **18**(1), 34–45.

Victor, M., Adams, R. D., & Collins, G. H. (1989). *The Wernicke–Korsakoff Syndrome and related Neurological Disorders of Alcoholism and Malnutrition*. Philadelphia: FA Davis Co.

Wernicke, C. (1881). *Lehrbuch Der Gehirnkrankheiten Für Aerzte Und Studirende*, Band II. Kassel: Fischer.

Wijnia, J. W. (2022). A Clinician's View of Wernicke–Korsakoff Syndrome. *Journal of Clinical Medicine*, **11**(22), 6755.

Wijnia, J. W., Oudman, E., van Gool, W. A., et al. (2016). Severe infections are common in thiamine deficiency and may be related to cognitive outcomes: a cohort study of 68 patients with Wernicke–Korsakoff syndrome. *Psychosomatics*, **57**(6), 624–633.

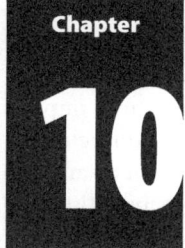

Cognitive Rehabilitation

The phrases 'cognitive stimulation', 'cognitive training', and 'cognitive rehabilitation' all feature in the literature on ageing and dementia. Whilst there is a degree of overlap between them, they have distinct meanings.

- **Cognitive stimulation** refers to any activity that makes use of cognitive function. The activity might not be primarily aimed at improving cognitive function and may also include physical activity and social interaction. Dance and Tai Chi classes would be examples of activities which involve all three components.
- **Cognitive rehabilitation** focusses on improving life skills in people who have experienced a decline in cognitive function. Common approaches include:
1. Cognitive training exercises, which involve practising specific cognitive skills, such as attention, memory, and problem solving, to improve these abilities over time. This can be done either with pencil-and-paper formats or computer-based exercises.
2. Compensation, which involves teaching and using alternative strategies to compensate for cognitive deficits, such as external memory aids, mnemonics, and breaking down complex tasks into smaller steps.
3. Environmental modification, which may include adapting the physical environment in a way that makes things easier for someone with cognitive deficits.

Although most cognitive rehabilitation techniques were developed for people with acquired brain injury, many of these techniques and principles have subsequently been applied with degenerative disorders (Clare & Woods, 2001).

The International Classification of Functioning, Disability and Health

To understand the aims of rehabilitation, the International Classification of Functioning, Disability and Health (ICF) is a useful framework, developed by the World Health Organization in 2001 to accompany the International Classification of Disease (ICD). The aim was to provide a framework for specifying how a particular illness might affect someone at the level of function. It distinguishes three levels of function:

1. **Impairment** refers to a problem in body function. This can be in relation to a physical, mental, or cognitive system.
2. **Activity** refers to the execution of a task or action. This would cover concepts such as activities of daily living, including washing, dressing, eating, and so forth.
3. **Participation** refers to a person's ability to engage in real-life experiences, such as work, recreation, and education.

One way to think about the difference between activity and participation might be that the former refers to interaction with the physical environment, whereas participation is concerned with the social environment. The different levels are inter-related, so that an impairment may limit someone's ability to perform an activity, which in turn impacts upon someone's ability to participate in society. For example, a memory *impairment* may reduce ability to engage in the *activity* of learning new information, which could be a barrier to *participating* in a course of study/education. The ultimate aim of cognitive rehabilitation is to maximise the ability to participate, often by working to make changes at the activity level.

Memory Rehabilitation

Memory is possibly the most widely investigated area of cognitive rehabilitation, and many of the techniques developed to assist with memory problems also have applications for rehabilitation of executive function (Wilson, 2009). The strategies used are often characterised as *internal*, which usually refers to strategies used by the individual, or *external*, which refers to the use of a device such as a diary, shopping list, or mobile phone. With both internal and external memory aids, the aim is not to improve people's memory at the impairment level, but to bring about improvement at the participation level by making changes at the activity level.

Internal Memory Strategies

This refers to strategies and principles people can use to improve their memory function. It includes the use of effective rehearsal strategies, mnemonics, errorless learning, and vanishing cues.

Rehearsal is a core element of internal memory strategies, but some rehearsal strategies are more effective than others. One of the fundamental distinctions is between active and passive rehearsal, where the former involves interacting with or manipulating the information in some way. For example, repeatedly reading a list of words would constitute passive rehearsal, whereas repeating a sequence of (1) reading the words, (2) covering them up, then (3) trying to recall them would constitute active rehearsal. Active rehearsal produces better results than passive rehearsal (Nairne, 1986). Another important factor is how the rehearsal is carried out over time, which gives rise to the distinction between massed and distributed practice (Ebbinghaus, 1885). Massed practice is done all at once, whereas distributed practice is spread out over a period of time. For example, if one hour were allocated to rehearsing material, ten minutes spread across six days would be more beneficial than concentrating the rehearsal into one hour on a single day. Additionally, this schedule is more effective if the time periods between rehearsal sessions are progressively lengthened, which is known as expanding rehearsal (Landauer & Bjork, 1978).

Mnemonics are a form of active rehearsal. Verbal mnemonics have a long history of being used in education for remembering lists or sequences, by encoding them verbally as something easier to remember such as a rhyme. An example would be 'divorced, beheaded, died, divorced, beheaded, survived' as way to remember the fates of King Henry VIII's wives by using a rhyme. 'Every Good Boy Deserves Favours' and FACE have been used to remember the notes associated with the lines and spaces of the treble clef in music. Another popular strategy for remembering lists/sequences is chunking (Miller, 1956), whereby a sequence is broken down into smaller groups of items. A shopping list can be made easier to remember by grouping the items into categories such as fruit, vegetables, bakery, meat, and so forth. Thus, bread, bananas, crumpets, carrots, fairy cakes, apples, chicken, aubergines, sausages, broccoli, grapes, and bacon would be best reorganised as {apples, bananas, grapes}, {aubergine, broccoli, carrots}, {bread, crumpets, fairy cakes}, and {chicken, bacon, and sausages}. Similarly, a string of digits such as 01753653892 is more easily remembered as 01753 65 38 92. Use of familiarity can also enhance encoding by associating the target item with something familiar – for example, remembering someone's name by linking it with someone already familiar to you: Charles → King; Humphrey → Bogart; Donald → duck.

Visual mnemonics refers to the use of visual imagery to facilitate encoding of information, as things are easier to remember if you can create a picture of them. For example, the method of loci consists of imagining a familiar route and creating an image of the items to be remembered at various places along the route. This technique is a favourite of people famous for demonstrating impressive feats of memory, including modern celebrities such as Derren Brown (Brown, 2006) and mnemonists such as Shereshevsky, studied over a 30-year period by Luria (1968).

Errorless learning is a principle rather than a technique, and has been applied widely in the rehabilitation of people with acquired brain injury (Wilson, Baddeley, & Evans, 1994). In contrast to trial-and-error learning, guessing is discouraged, and mistakes are immediately corrected when material is being learned. The rationale is that if people make mistakes, they are subsequently more likely to remember those mistakes than the correct answers/responses. This is often used in conjunction with the technique of vanishing cues (Glisky, Schacter, & Tulving, 1986), an example of which would be to present a list of words to learn, and then present partial words as cues during recall, gradually reducing the number of letters with subsequent trials. A meta-analysis of studies concluded that whilst errorless learning was effective, vanishing cues only had a small effect (Kessels & Haan, 2003). A major difficulty with using vanishing cues is that performance drops markedly with the removal of the final cue (Wilson, 2009), making its use in clinical practice limited.

Internal memory strategies have been shown to be effective in the general population, and in a range of patients with memory disorders. There is also a significant literature base specifically addressing their use in patients with dementia.

External Memory Aids

Whereas internal memory aids are strategies which allow people to make more effective use of the memory ability they have, external memory aids are devices you use to compensate for the limitations of your memory. This can take the form of traditional pen and paper aids, such as diaries and notebooks, or more modern technology such as mobile phones. It is worth noting that external memory aids are used extensively by people without neurological impairment, with lists, notes, and calendars being the most popular (Wilson, 2009). One thing to bear in mind when choosing which external aids to try is that people are most likely to be successful with something they have used prior to the onset of dementia. For example, if someone is used to using a paper diary before they developed dementia, this would be a good place to start; if someone has never used electronic reminders, this would be more difficult.

The use of external memory aids overlaps with environmental modification, as strategies such as Post-it notes, whiteboards, calendars, and alarms can be applied within the home. Portable memory aids such as shopping list, pagers, and satellite navigation can be extremely effective at facilitating function outside the home. Whilst separate items can be used, many forms of memory aid are now incorporated into modern mobile phones.

Cognitive Training Exercises

Cognitive training aims to improve areas of cognitive function by using repeated practice of tasks targeting specific cognitive abilities such as working memory, attention, problem solving, and processing speed. Some of the literature on cognitive training conflates repetitive exercises with training in the use of applied memory strategies (e.g. mnemonics, visual imagery) (Mowszowski, Batchelor, & Naismith, 2010), whereas it could be argued that the latter is really a form of compensation. For example, the ACTIVE study (Advanced Cognitive Training for Independent and Vital Elderly) looked at cognitive training in three areas: (1) memory, (2) inductive reasoning, and (3) processing speed (Rebok et al., 2014). The training received by the memory group was in fact instruction and practice in the use of internal memory strategies. This study excluded individuals with dementia, although their cut-off criteria (a score of <23 on the MMSE) may have included individuals with MCI. They found a beneficial effect of training was still apparent after 10 years for the reasoning and processing speed groups, but not for the memory group. Gates et al. (2011) reviewed the evidence for cognitive training in MCI. They concluded there was little evidence for the efficacy of memory training in MCI, although cognitive training in multiple cognitive domains was more effective. There was greater evidence for the efficacy of cognitive exercise than memory strategy training, although this may have been due to studies on cognitive exercise using higher training volumes.

The format of cognitive training exercise had traditionally been based around pen-and-paper tasks, but in recent decades there has been a large growth in the use of computerised training exercises and games (Gates & Valenzuela, 2010; Zhang et al., 2019). Hill et al. (2017) reviewed studies on computerised training in MCI and dementia. They concluded there was evidence for mild to moderate effects in MCI, but only weak evidence for efficacy in dementia, which came from three studies using immersive technology such as virtual reality.

Environmental Modification

Environmental modification for older adults, both with and without cognitive impairment, has been widely investigated from different angles. These include physical adaptations to prevent falls (Guo et al., 2013) and adaptive technologies such as reminder systems and safety sensors (Lauriks et al., 2007). Whilst still carried out within the format of an MDT, environmental modification is more commonly the remit of occupational therapy (Padilla et al., 2011).

Evidence for the Effectiveness of Cognitive Rehabilitation with Dementia

Amieva et al. (2016) randomised 653 patients with a diagnosis of Alzheimer's disease to one of three groups: cognitive training, reminiscence therapy (cognitive stimulation), or individualised cognitive rehabilitation. Over a follow-up period of two years, they found cognitive rehabilitation was associated with a lower level of functional disability and a six-month delay before institutionalisation was required. They did not find evidence for an effect of cognitive training or reminiscence therapy. A similar result was found in a Cochrane review of 11 trials of cognitive training and 1 trial of cognitive rehabilitation (Baher-Fuchs, Clare, & Woods, 2013), with only the trial of cognitive rehabilitation showing any benefits (Claire et al., 2010).

Cognitive Training in Healthy Older Adults, MCI, and Dementia

Other reviews looking at cognitive training have reported mixed results, which may be related to factors such as study design, the stage of cognitive impairment, or the choice of outcome measure. With the example of cognitive training exercises, reviews have suggested cognitive training may be most beneficial with healthy older adults (Gates & Valenzuela, 2010), moderately beneficial in people with MCI (Gates et al., 2011; Zhang et al., 2019), and of least benefit in people with dementia (Huntley et al. 2015).

The choice of outcome measures used in studies needs to be considered carefully, as impressive results are sometimes claimed when the outcome measure is performance on the task on which the training was undertaken, but with no evidence of a general improvement in cognitive ability outside of that task. This was illustrated by Owen et al. (2010), who looked at the effects of a 6-week computerised training programme on the cognitive abilities of 11,430 healthy participants. The tasks were aimed at improving reasoning, memory, planning, visuospatial skills, and attention. Although improvements were seen in all of the trained tasks, there was no evidence of generalisation outside of these task – that is, the improvement seen after training on the memory task did not improve any aspects of memory function other than performing that specific task.

Whilst there is some evidence that cognitive training can lead to an improvement in cognitive function, it is important to note that there is currently no evidence to indicate that this can lead to a reduction in dementia prevalence (Zhang et al., 2019).

Cognitive Stimulation

Claire and Woods (2004) defined cognitive stimulation as engaging in a 'range of activities and discussions aimed at general enhancement of cognitive and social function'. This is aimed at people with dementia, the earliest example being reality orientation (Taulbee & Folsom, 1966). Aguirre, Woods, Spector, and Orrell (2013) reviewed 15 studies on cognitive stimulation and found benefits to cognition and self-rated quality of life. Spector et al. (2003) carried out a randomised control trial on 201 older adults with dementia and reported improvement on the MMSE, the ADAS-COG, and the Quality-of-Life Alzheimer's Disease scale. The degree of improvement was reported as comparable to that seen with AChE medication.

Evidence for the Effectiveness of Environmental Modification

Gitlin, Lieber, and Lararine (2003) reviewed 63 studies looking at environmental modification in different situations. Their conclusion was that 90% of studies reported positive results, but generalisability was limited by small sample sizes and the majority being based in nursing homes. Large-scale studies of environmental modification are lacking, which possibly reflects the difficulty in carrying them out and the probable need for studies based across multiple sites.

Things to Bear in Mind When Considering the Evidence

'Absence of evidence is not evidence of absence' is a quote associated with cosmologist Carl Sagan (1977), but traceable in various forms to earlier sources (Quoteinvestigator.com, n.d.). It seems highly applicable to the study of cognitive rehabilitation in dementia and

MCI, where the emerging evidence base may seem to deliver contradictory results. Whilst large-scale reviews and meta-analyses might be considered the gold standard for reliable evaluation of evidence, they are always limited by the quality of the evidence available. Differences in methodology, terminology, and choice of outcome measure can rapidly reduce the number of individual studies which can be included, which in turn limits the conclusions which can be drawn. Large-scale studies are difficult to carry out in practice. It is important to bear in mind that there can be a large number of reasons why it has not been possible to demonstrate the effectiveness of a particular intervention other than the intervention not being effective.

It is equally important to consider the quality of the evidence in favour of something working. As mentioned earlier, claims for a particular training programme being effective must be considered in the context of what 'effective' means. For improvement in cognitive ability to be meaningful, the evidence must demonstrate something over and above increased performance on a specific training task; ideally, it should translate into an improvement in real-world function. Here it is important to remember the difference between a result which is statistically significant and one which is clinically significant. Statistical significance is an indication of reliability (i.e. how likely is it that the difference you have observed did not occur by chance). An effect may be highly reliable, as in most people show the effect, but still be quite small and not big enough to make any difference in real life. It is also necessary to consider the relationship between statistical significance, effect size, and sample size. Statistical significance is related to sample size, so the more participants you include in a study the greater the chance of a significant result. With a small sample an intervention would need to make a much bigger difference to be significant, whereas with a very large sample size even a small (but reliable) difference would be significant. With the increased availability of online training programmes, it is possible to get access to very large numbers of participants, so considering the effect size becomes highly important. (See Owen et al. (2010) for a discussion about statistical significance and effect size in relation to computerised cognitive training.)

Key Points

- Cognitive rehabilitation is aimed at improving the function of people who have experienced cognitive decline.
- The most common methods for achieving this include cognitive training, compensation, and environmental modification.
- Cognitive stimulation refers to any activity which engages cognitive processes, but may not specifically be intended to improve cognitive function.
- The most common framework in which rehabilitation is conducted is the WHO's International Classification of Functioning, Disability and Health. This distinguishes between impairment, activity limitation, and participation restriction. Rehabilitation is generally aimed at increasing participation.
- Evidence for the effectiveness of cognitive rehabilitation can be slightly contradictory, as some studies are limited by small sample sizes. Meta-analyses are limited by the availability of studies which meet their inclusion criteria.
- A multi-component rehabilitation package tailored to the individual is likely to be most successful.

References

Aguirre, E., Woods, R. T., Spector, A., & Orrell, M. (2013). Cognitive stimulation for dementia: A systematic review of the evidence of effectiveness from randomised controlled trials. *Ageing Research Reviews*, **12**(1), 253–62.

Amieva, H., Robert, P. H., Grandoulier, A. S., et al. (2016). Group and individual cognitive therapies in Alzheimer's disease: The ETNA3 randomized trial. *International Psychogeriatrics*, **28**(5), 707–17.

Baher-Fuchs, A., Clare, L., & Woods, B. (2013). Cognitive training and cognitive rehabilitation for mild to moderate Alzheimer's disease and vascular dementia. *Cochrane Database of Systematic Reviews*, 6: CD003260.

Brown, D. (2006). *Tricks of the Mind*. London: Transworld Publishers.

Clare, L., & Woods, B. (2001). A role for cognitive rehabilitation in dementia care. *Neuropsychological Rehabilitation*, **11**(3–4), 193–6.

Clare, L., & Woods, R. T. (2004). Cognitive training and cognitive rehabilitation for people with early-stage Alzheimer's disease: A review. *Neuropsychological Rehabilitation*, **14**(4), 385–401.

Clare, L., Linden, D. E., Woods, R. T., et al. (2010). Goal-oriented cognitive rehabilitation for people with early-stage Alzheimer disease: A single-blind randomized controlled trial of clinical efficacy. *The American Journal of Geriatric Psychiatry*, **18**(10), 928–39.

Ebbinghaus, H. (1885). *Memory: A Contribution to Experimental Psychology*. New York: Dover.

Gates, N., Sachdev, P., Fiatarone Singh, M. & Valenzuela, M. (2011). Cognitive and memory training in adults at risk of dementia: A systematic review. *BMC Geriatrics*, **11**(1), 1–14.

Gates, N., & Valenzuela, M. (2010). Cognitive exercise and its role in cognitive function in older adults. *Current Psychiatry Reports*, **12**, 20–7.

Gitlin, L. N., Liebman, J., & Winter, L. (2003). Are environmental interventions effective in the management of Alzheimer's disease and related disorders? A synthesis of the evidence. *Alzheimer's Care Today*, **4**(2), 85–107.

Glisky, E. L., Schacter, D. L., & Tulving, E. (1986). Learning and retention of computer-related vocabulary in memory-impaired patients: Method of vanishing cues. *Journal of Clinical and Experimental Neuropsychology*, **8**(3), 292–312.

Guo, J. L., Tsai, Y. Y., Liao, J. Y., Tu, H. M., & Huang, C. M. (2014). Interventions to reduce the number of falls among older adults with/without cognitive impairment: an exploratory meta-analysis. *International Journal of Geriatric Psychiatry*, **29**(7), 661–9.

Hill, N. T., Mowszowski, L., Naismith, S. L., et al. (2017). Computerized cognitive training in older adults with mild cognitive impairment or dementia: A systematic review and meta-analysis. *American Journal of Psychiatry*, **174**(4), 329–40.

Huntley, J. D., Gould, R. L., Liu, K., Smith, M., & Howard, R. J. (2015). Do cognitive interventions improve general cognition in dementia? A meta-analysis and meta-regression. *BMJ Open*, **5**(4), e005247.

Kessels, R. P., & Haan, E. H. (2003). Implicit learning in memory rehabilitation: A meta-analysis on errorless learning and vanishing cues methods. *Journal of Clinical and Experimental Neuropsychology*, **25**(6), 805–14.

Landauer, T. K., & Bjork, R. A. (1978). Optimal rehearsal patterns and name learning. In M. M. Gruneberg, P. E. Morris, & R. N. Sykes (Eds.), *Practical Aspects of Memory* (pp. 625–632). London: Academic Press.

Lauriks, S., Reinersmann, A., Van der Roest, H. G., et al. (2007). Review of ICT-based services for identified unmet needs in people with dementia. *Ageing Research Reviews*, **6**(3), 223–46.

Luria, A. (1968). *Mind of a Mnemonist*. Cambridge, MA; Harvard University Press.

Miller, G. A. (1956). The magical number seven plus or minus two: Some limits on our capacity for processing information. *Psychological Review*, **63**, 81–97.

Mowszowski, L., Batchelor, J., & Naismith, S. L. (2010). Early intervention for cognitive decline: Can cognitive training be used as a selective prevention technique? *International Psychogeriatrics*, **22**(4), 537–48.

Nairne, J. S. (1986). Active and passive processing during primary rehearsal. The American Journal of Psychology, **99**(3), 301–14.

Owen, A. M., Hampshire, A., Grahn, J. A., et al. (2010). Putting brain training to the test. *Nature*, **465**(7299), 775–8.

Padilla, R. (2011). Effectiveness of interventions designed to modify the activity demands of the occupations of self-care and leisure for people with Alzheimer's disease and related dementias. *The American Journal of Occupational Therapy*, **65**(5), 523–31.

Quoteinvestigator.com. (n.d.). Absence of evidence is not evidence of absence. https://quoteinvestigator.com/2019/09/17/absence/#f+436457+1+10.

Rebok, G. W., Ball, K., Guey, L. T., et al. (2014). Ten-year effects of the ACTIVE cognitive training trial on cognition and everyday functioning in older adults. *Journal of the American Geriatrics Society*, **62**(1), 16–24.

Sagan, C. (1977). *The Dragons of Eden: Speculations on the Evolution of Human Intelligence*. New York; Random House.

Spector, A., Thorgrimsen, L., Woods, B., et al. (2003). Efficacy of an evidence-based cognitive stimulation therapy programme for people with dementia: Randomised controlled trial. *The British Journal of Psychiatry*, **183**(3), 248–54.

Taulbee, L. R., & Folsom, J. C. (1966). Reality orientation for geriatric patients. *Psychiatric Services*, **17**(5), 133–5.

Wilson, B. (2009). *Memory Rehabilitation: Integrating Theory and Practice*. New York: The Guilford Press.

Wilson, B. A., Baddeley, A., Evans, J., & Shiel, A. (1994). Errorless learning in the rehabilitation of memory impaired people. *Neuropsychological Rehabilitation*, **4**(3), 307–26.

Zhang, H., Huntley, J., Bhome, R. et al. (2019). Effect of computerised cognitive training on cognitive outcomes in mild cognitive impairment: A systematic review and meta-analysis. *BMJ Open*, **9**(8), e027062.

Pharmacological Interventions

Developing pharmacological interventions for dementia has proved challenging. Although there have been a large number of clinical trials of potential treatments, 99.6% have been unsuccessful (Cummings, Morstorf, & Zhong, 2014), and no new drugs for dementia have been licensed in the UK since memantine in 2003. In addition, currently available 'anti-dementia' drugs are associated with relatively modest temporary improvements in cognitive ability (Buckley & Saltpeter, 2015) and large placebo effects (Fink et al., 2020). Despite disappointing progress in the area of pharmacological interventions, there are new treatments in development. Most research has focussed on Alzheimer's disease.

Before looking at the results of clinical trials, it is worth considering the difference between efficacy and effectiveness. Efficacy refers to the ability of a drug/intervention to produce a demonstrable effect under tightly controlled conditions. This is usually what is studied in randomised control trials. Effectiveness is the degree to which an intervention helps people. It is possible to have evidence for the efficacy of a particular drug which is unfortunately not accompanied by a demonstration of effectiveness – that is, it does not make a difference in real life.

The Difference Between Disease-Modifying and Symptom-Modifying Treatments

There are two types of pharmacological intervention, with different aims. A disease-modifying treatment targets the underlying disease process (or at least one of them, if there are several), with the aim of halting or even reversing the effects. This would be the ultimate aim of pharmacological treatment of dementia, and a number of drugs have been developed with the intention of stopping and potentially reversing the development of toxic proteins such as beta amyloid. At the time of writing, there are no disease-modifying drugs for dementia licensed for use in the UK. The Food and Drug Administration (FDA) in America has recently licensed aducanumab, a monoclonal antibody therapy, for use. This has not been without controversy and questions have been raised regarding whether there is sufficient evidence in relation to the efficacy and possible side effects to justify this (Walsh et al., 2021).

A symptom-modifying treatment does not affect the course of the underlying disease. Its effect is to produce some form of symptomatic improvement. There are currently four symptom-modifying drugs available in the UK: three acetylcholinesterase inhibitors, recommended for mild to moderate Alzheimer's disease (AD), and memantine, an MDMA receptor antagonist, recommended for moderate to severe AD (Thomas & Grossberg, 2009).

Acetylcholinesterase Inhibitors

Acetyl choline (ACh) is a neurotransmitter. When an action potential (electrical impulse) is generated by a neuron, it travels along the axon and reaches a chemical junction known as a synapse which links to the dendrite of another neuron (see Figure 11.1). When the action potential arrives at the synapse, a neurotransmitter is released, which moves across the synaptic gap and activates a receptor on the next neuron to which it is connected. This alters the resting membrane potential of that neuron, known as the post-synaptic membrane. If the collective activity from connected neurons raises this to a certain level, the cell fires its own action potential. Once this happens, the neurotransmitter must be removed from the receptor. The removal of acetyl choline is achieved by the release of an enzyme, which breaks the acetyl choline down to choline and acetic acid. This terminates the effect on the receptor and prevents the ACh activating other receptors (McHardy et al., 2017). There are

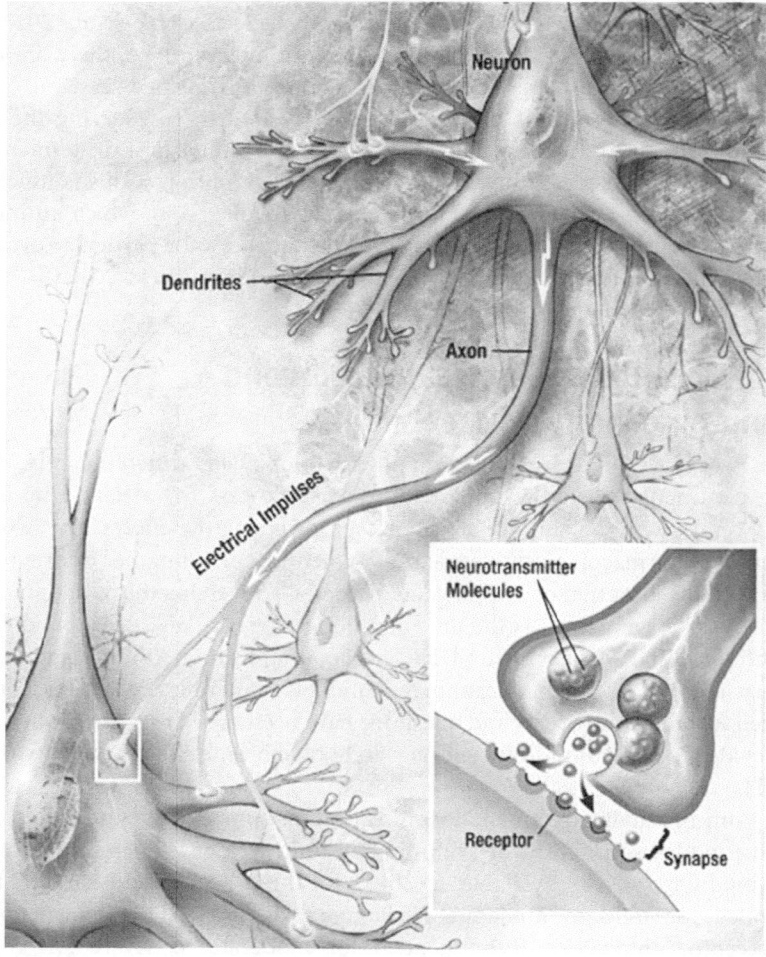

Figure 11.1 Illustration of neuron and synapse. Chemical synapse schema cropped © National Institute on Aging (https://commons.wikimedia.Org/wiki/File:Chemical_synapse_schema_cropped.jpg). Public domain.

two main types of enzyme carrying out this role: acetylcholinesterase (AchE), located in the synaptic cleft and synaptic membrane, and butyrylcholinesterase (BuChE) which is associated with glial cells (Giacobini, 2001). AchE is the main target for intervention as it is the predominant form of cholinesterase enzyme in the brains of healthy people (Nordberg et al., 2013).

AchE inhibitors exert an effect by reducing the activity of the cholinesterase enzymes, which raises the level of available ACh and increases the duration of its action (Colovic et al., 2013).

There are currently three AchE inhibitors licensed for use in the UK and recommended for mild to moderate AD: donepezil, galantamine, and rivastigmine (National Institute for Health and Care Excellence (NICE), 2018). Rivastigmine differs from the other two as it is both an AchE and a BuChE inhibitor (Nordberg et al., 2013). Tacrine, the first AchE inhibitor to be licensed, was withdrawn in 2013 due to a lack of evidence for its effectiveness and a poor side-effect profile (Marucci et al., 2021). The rationale for using AchE inhibitors was that AD results in degeneration of neural pathways which utilise Ach, therefore increasing the availability of Ach may produce some symptomatic improvement.

The Evidence for AchE Inhibitors

Effectiveness

The first problem with these medications is the evidence for their effectiveness, and relatively small clinical benefits (Grossberg, 2003). Buckley and Salpeter (2015) conducted a systematic review of the evidence which covered 257 studies. They concluded that there is no evidence for the effectiveness of these drugs in patients with advanced disease, vascular dementia, or aged over 85. There was evidence for small, improvements in cognition and function in early AD and Lewy body dementia, but it was uncertain whether these changes would make a difference clinically. Any benefits observed were temporary and described as 'minimal' after a year.

The outcome measures used in clinical trails have tended to be global measures of cognition, rather than using more detailed neuropsychological assessment. The gold standard cognitive measure for clinical trials has been the Alzheimer's Disease (AD) Assessment Scale-Cognitive Subscale (ADAS-Cog) (Rosen, Mohs, & Davis, 1984), which has item scores ranging from 1 to 5, and a total score from 0 to 70. An increase of 4 points is considered a positive result. A reduction of 6 points a year is considered typical progression (Ito et al., 2010). The other popular measure has been the Mini-Mental Status Examination (MMSE) (Folstein et al., 1975), which is a 30-item screening instrument. Knight et al. (2018) carried out a meta-analysis on 80 clinical trials using aChE inhibitors or memantine which used the MMSE as outcome measure, and reported an average advantage of approximately one point when comparing the treatment conditions to controls.

It is worth emphasising the difference between statistical significance and clinical significance. Statistical significance tells you whether a result is reliable, as in it did not happen by chance. If a result is statistically significant in a drug trial, it means people in the treatment group consistently did better than people in the control group, even if the difference was not very large. To be clinically significant, the treatment would need to make a difference to the person's function or well-being. It is therefore possible that an intervention may be statistically significant, but not clinically significant because whatever change occurred did not make a difference to the person's everyday function or well-being.

Side Effects

As it is not possible to limit the effects of aChE inhibitors to specific areas of the body, their use will affect levels of aCh throughout. Common side effects reported include issues with the digestive tract, such as nausea, vomiting, diarrhoea, abdominal pain, and loss of appetite. Insomnia, headaches, bradycardia, syncope, and muscle cramps are also reported (Moreta et al., 2021). The lack of evidence for effectiveness, combined with the accompanying side-effect profile, led to funding for these drugs being withdrawn in France (Rédaction, 2018) and temporarily withdrawn in England and Wales (NICE, 2009).

Placebo Effects

Placebo effects in clinical trials of aChE inhibitors have been frequently reported. In a review of 14 trials using the ADAS-cog as outcome measure, Kaduszkiewicz et al. (2005) reported that 12 studies showed a difference between treatment and placebo groups. However, the differences were relatively small, ranging from 1.3 to 3.9, which are below the recommended cut-off of 4 points. Whilst some trials have reported placebo effects to fade by week 6 (Lockwood et al., 2006), Ito et al. (2010) reported a peak placebo effect around 11 weeks, which did not fade until approximately a year.

Nursing Home Care

It is often cited that the use of aChE inhibitors in more advanced dementia delays the need for nursing home care by several months. Although this appears to have entered conventional wisdom, the evidence to support it is not particularly strong. Courtney et al. (2004) carried out a randomised control trial investigating this in relation to donepezil and did not find an effect. Other studies which have reported a delay in people using various different forms of medication, including memantine, typically lacked randomisation, placebo conditions, or blinding (Karlawish, 2004; Schneider & Oizilbash, 2004). Howard et al. (2015) conducted a randomised, double blind, placebo-controlled trial looking at the use of memantine and donepezil, following up with participants over a period of four years. They reported that discontinuation of donepezil in the first year of treatment doubled the risk of requiring a nursing home placement. This was not seen at follow-up points after this, and the addition of memantine did not make a difference.

aChE Inhibitors and Non-Alzheimer's Dementia

Given the mode of action of aChE inhibitors and the rationale for their use in AD, it might be expected that their potential for a therapeutic effect would be greatest in types of dementia associated with cholinergic depletion, but not in types of dementia where cholinergic pathways are thought to be less affected. Consequently, patients with FTD would not be expected to benefit from this type of medication, and indeed no benefits have been found (Gazzina et al., 2017). Pure vascular dementia is not considered to benefit from the use of these medications; however, the British Association for Psychopharmacology recommended their use in mixed dementia (O'Brien et al., 2017). Matsunaga et al. (2016) carried out a meta-analysis on the effects of aChE inhibitors in Lewy body disorders (Parkinson's disease, Parkinson's dementia, and DLB), concluding that they can be effective without interfering with motor function. Donepizil had the strongest evidence for improving cognition, whereas rivastigmine was most effective for behavioural disturbances. Galantamine showed no benefit over placebo.

Memantine

The last new drug to be licensed in the UK for symptomatic treatment of dementia was memantine, which has a different mechanism to the aChE inhibitors as it is a N-methyl-D-aspartate (NMDA) receptor antagonist. NMDA receptors are activated by the neurotransmitter glutamate, which is typically excitatory. An antagonist is a substance that binds to a receptor and decreases the effect of a neurotransmitter, whereas an agonist mimics the effect of the neurotransmitter and increases the effect. Memantine binds with NMDA receptors and reduces the excitatory effect of glutamate, an excess of which is thought to be toxic to neurons (Lipton, 2005). In their Cochrane review, McShane et al. (2019) concluded that there was evidence for a small benefit of memantine in moderate to severe AD, but no evidence of any benefit in mild AD. Although there have been suggestions that memantine may have a neuroprotective effect, it is not considered to be a disease-modifying drug (Thomas & Grossberg, 2009). O'Brien et al. (2017) recommended that memantine could be used in conjunction with an aChE inhibitor.

Disease-Modifying Drugs

Cummings and Fox (2017) considered the requirements for a disease-modifying therapy:

1. The definition of disease should include preclinical states, identified via biomarkers or a decline in cognitive function which does not meet the criteria for dementia. This is probably the stage at which disease-modifying therapies will be most effective, by concentrating on prevention.
2. Modifying means there is a change in the clinical course of the disease because of a change in the underlying disease process.
3. Therapy refers to a structured intervention, which may be pharmacological or non-pharmacological.

A number of different classes of disease-modifying drugs have been investigated and thought to show potential in animal-based studies but have yet to demonstrate efficacy in clinical trials. The main strategy has been to try to stop the development of beta amyloid protein, or even to remove existing accumulations. Whilst some drugs have demonstrated at post-mortem examination that beta amyloid load was lessened when compared to controls, this did not correspond to any detectable benefit for the patients (Holmes et al., 2008). The main classes of drug being investigated are: β-secretase and γ-secretase inhibitors, vaccinations, passive immunisation, and anti-tau strategies (Ghezzi, Scarpini, & Galimberti, 2013).

Although no disease-modifying drugs have been licensed for use in the UK, aducanamab has been licensed for use in America. The mode of action for this drug, and the evidence for its effectiveness, will be briefly reviewed.

Mode of Action

Aducanamab is a monoclonal antibody therapy, which is a class of drugs modelled on the function of the immune system. The immune system creates blood proteins called antibodies in response to detecting a toxin or other foreign substance (antigen).

The monoclonal antibody therapies are created to target specific cells which have biological markers, potentially reducing off-target effects and side effects and increasing efficacy (Castelli, McGonigle, & Hornby, 2019). Aducanamab is designed to target and remove beta amyloid protein from the brains of people with AD, and evidence from studies using PET scans to measure amyloid load suggests it is effective at doing this. According to the amyloid cascade hypothesis, this should be accompanied by some clinical benefit such as improvement of cognitive symptoms, or at least a halting of disease progression. However, strong evidence for this has not emerged, as two randomised phase III clinical trials have shown conflicting results (Lalli et al., 2021), and the clinical relevance of the effects demonstrated has been questioned (Lui, Schneider, & Howard, 2021). A stage IV clinical trial has been set up for aducanumab with the aim of completing in 2030 (Castelli, McGonigle, & Hornby, 2019), which is a large-scale evaluation carried out over a number of years after the drug has initially been licensed.

At the time of writing, another monoclonal antibody therapy called donanemab had gained a lot of media attention. Sims et al. (2023) reported a large-scale multi-centre trial involving an infusion of donanemab or placebo every 4 weeks over a period of 72 weeks. The level of beta amyloid and tau protein was monitored by PET scan, and cognitive functional change was measured with integrated Alzheimer's Disease Rating Scale (iADRS) (Wessels et al., 2015). The findings were that patients in the donanemab arm showed reduced amyloid load when compared to the placebo arm, and even complete amyloid clearance in patients who had a lower load to begin with. There was no significant difference apparent on tau PET scans between donanemab and controls. On the iADRS, neither group showed improvement in cognition or function, and both groups continued to decline. However, for patients with low/medium levels of tau pathology, the donanemab arm showed a least-squares mean decline of 6.02, compared to 9.27 in the control group – a difference of 35.1%. For patients with higher levels of tau pathology, smaller differences were seen.

Plaques, Tangles, and Amyloid Oligomers

Although attention has focussed on insoluble forms of amyloid such as that found in plaques, evidence has accumulated that a soluble form of amyloid found in amyloid oligomers is the form associated with neurotoxicity and progression of AD (Gaspar et al., 2010; Yang et al., 2017). Tau protein accumulates in the form of tangles, which form within neurons, and is concentrated in the medial temporal areas. A longitudinal PET study looking at tau and amyloid indicated that tau protein only begins to accumulate outside of the medial temporal areas once amyloid load has reached a critical threshold level (Hanseeuw et al., 2019). There is evidence to suggest beta amyloid accumulation may progress for up to 13 years before tau begins to build up (Therneau et al., 2021). Once beta amyloid has reached a certain level, it initiates a chain of events which continue even if the amyloid level is subsequently reduced. The window of opportunity for pharmacological intervention to reduce beta amyloid load is therefore likely to be during the period before it has led to a rise in levels of tau.

Key Points

- Most of the development of pharmacological treatment of dementia has concentrated on AD.
- Although a lot of resources have been committed to this area of research, very few treatments have been developed. More than 99% of clinical trials have been unsuccessful.
- Treatments can be divided into symptom modification and disease modification. Initial research concentrated on symptom modification, and there are currently four medications licensed for this purpose.
- Although clinical trials show some evidence for the efficacy of these drugs, the effects tend to be quite small and the degree to which they produce clinical benefit is questionable.
- Several classes of drugs have been investigated, usually with a mode of action intended to reduce levels of amyloid protein, but none have been licensed for the use in the UK, and only one for use in America.
- Whilst biomarker studies have shown that the level of amyloid protein can be reduced (efficacy), there is a lack of strong evidence that this translates into clinical benefits (effectiveness).

Appendix K Types of Clinical Trial

Initial research on drugs is usually laboratory-based and tested with animal studies. This in itself is not sufficient, as different species have different metabolisms and effects seen in animals may not be transferrable to humans. Once the development of a drug moves onto the stage of testing in humans, this is referred to as a clinical trial. There are generally considered to be four types of clinical trial. The following definitions are taken from the World Health Organization (WHO, 2022):

- Phase I studies attempt to establish the safe dose range and potential side effects in a small group of people.
- Phase II studies again focus on side effects but use a larger group of people than a Phase I trial. The efficacy of a drug is usually also evaluated to some extent during this phase.
- Phase III studies are larger, multi-centre studies which look at efficacy and safety over a longer period, usually 6–12 months. These should be randomised control trials.
- Phase IV studies take place once a drug has been approved, and take place over a longer time frame, usually several years.

References

Buckley, J., & Saltpeter, S. (2015). A risk-benefit assessment of dementia medications: Systematic review of the evidence. *Drugs and Ageing*, **32**(6), 453–67.

Castelli, M. S., McGonigle, P., & Hornby, P. J. (2019). The pharmacology and therapeutic applications of monoclonal antibodies. *Pharmacology Research & Perspectives*, **7**(6), e00535.

Colovic, M. B., Krstic, D. Z., Lazarevic-Pasti, T. D., Bondzic, A. M., & Vasic, V. M. (2013). Acetylcholinesterase inhibitors: Pharmacology and toxicology. *Current Neuropharmacology*, **11**(3), 315–35.

Cummings, J. L., Morstorf, T., & Zhong, K. (2014). Alzheimer's disease drug-development pipeline: Few candidates, frequent failures. *Alzheimer's Research & Therapy*, **6**(4), 1–7.

Cummings, J. L., & Fox, N. (2017). Defining disease modifying therapy for Alzheimer's disease. *Journal of Prevention of Alzheimer's Disease*, **4**(2), 109–15.

Fink, H. A., Linskens, E. J., MacDonald, R., et al. (2020). Benefits and harms of prescription drugs and supplements for treatment of clinical Alzheimer-type dementia: A systematic review and meta-analysis. *Annals of Internal Medicine*, **172**(10), 656–68.

Folstein, M., Folsten, S., & McHugh, P. (1975). Mini-mental state: a practical method for grading the cognitive state of patients for the clinician. *Journal of Psychiatry Research*, **12**, 189–98.

Gaspar, R. C., Villarreal, S. A., Bowles, N., et al. (2010). Oligomers of beta-amyloid are sequestered into and seed new plaques in the brains of an AD mouse model. *Experimental Neurology*, **223**(2), 394–400.

Gazzina, S., Manes, M. A., Padovani, A., & Borroni, B. (2017). Clinical and biological phenotypes of frontotemporal dementia: Perspectives for disease modifying therapies. *European Journal of Pharmacology*, **817**, 76–85.

Ghezzi, L., Scarpini, E., & Galimberti, D. (2013). Disease-modifying drugs in Alzheimer's disease. *Drug Design, Development and Therapy*, 1471–9.

Giacobinni, E. (2001). Selective inhibitors of butyrylcholinesterase: A valid alternative for therapy of Alzheimer's disease. *Drugs and Ageing*, **18**, 891–8.

Grossberg, G. T. (2003). Cholinesterase inhibitors for the treatment of Alzheimer's disease: Getting on and staying on. *Current Therapeutic Research*, **64**(4), 216–35.

Hanseeuw, B. J., Betensky, R. A., Jacobs, H. I., et al. (2019). Association of amyloid and tau with cognition in preclinical Alzheimer disease: A longitudinal study. *JAMA Neurology*, **76**(8), 915–24.

Holmes, C., Boche, D., Wilkinson, D., et al. (2008). Long-term effects of Aβ42 immunisation in Alzheimer's disease: Follow-up of a randomised, placebo-controlled phase I trial. *The Lancet*, **372** (9634), 216–23.

Howard, R., McShane, R., Lindesay, J., et al. (2015). Nursing home placement in the Donepezil and Memantine in Moderate to Severe Alzheimer's Disease (DOMINO-AD) trial: Secondary and post-hoc analyses. *The Lancet Neurology*, **14**(12), 1171–1181.

Ito, K., Ahadieh, S., Corrigan, B., et al. (2010). Disease progression meta-analysis model in Alzheimer's disease. *Alzheimer's & Dementia*, **6**(1), 39–53.

Kaduszkiewicz, H., Zimmermann, T., Beck-Bornholdt, H. P., & van den Bussche, H. (2005). Cholinesterase inhibitors for patients with Alzheimer's disease: Systematic review of randomised clinical trials. *British Medical Journal*, **331**(7512), 321–7.

Karlawish, J. H. (2004). Donepezil delay to nursing home placement study is flawed. *Journal of the American Geriatric Society*, **52**, 845

Knight, R., Khondoker, M., Magill, N., Stewart, R., & Landau, S. (2018). A systematic review and meta-analysis of the effectiveness of acetylcholinesterase inhibitors and memantine in treating the cognitive symptoms of dementia. *Dementia and Geriatric Cognitive Disorders*, **45**(3–4), 131–51.

Lalli, G., Schott, J. M., Hardy, J., & De Strooper, B. (2021). Aducanumab: A new phase in therapeutic development for Alzheimer's disease?. *EMBO Molecular Medicine*, **13**(8), e14781.

Lipton, S. A. (2005). The molecular basis of memantine action in Alzheimer's disease and other neurologic disorders: Low-affinity, uncompetitive antagonism. *Current Alzheimer Research*, **2**(2), 155–65.

Liu, K. Y., Schneider, L. S., & Howard, R. (2021) The need to show minimum clinically important differences in Alzheimer's disease trials. *Lancet Psychiatry*, **8**(11), 1013–16.

Lockwood, P., Ewy, W., Hermann, D., & Holford, N. (2006). Application of clinical trial simulation to compare proof-of-concept study designs for drugs with a slow onset of effect: An example in Alzheimer's disease. *Pharmaceutical Research*, **23**(9), 2050–9.

Matsunaga, S., Kishi, T., Yasue, I., & Iwata, N. (2016). Cholinesterase inhibitors for Lewy body disorders: A meta-analysis. *International Journal of Neuropsychopharmacology*, **19**(2), 1–15.

McHardy, S. F., Wang, H. Y. L., McCowen, S. V., & Valdez, M. C. (2017). Recent advances in acetylcholinesterase inhibitors and reactivators: An update on the patent literature (2012–2015). *Expert Opinion on Therapeutic Patents*, **27**(4), 455–76.

McShane, R., Westby, M. J., & Roberts, E. (2019). Memantine for dementia. *Cochrane Database Syst Rev*. 2019 Mar 20; 3(3): CD003154.

Moreta, M. P. G., Burgos-Alonso, N., Torrecilla, M., Marco-Contelles, J., & Bruzos-Cidón, C. (2021). Efficacy of acetylcholinesterase inhibitors on cognitive function in Alzheimer's disease. *Review of Reviews. Biomedicines*, **9**(11), 1689.

National Institute for Health and Care Excellence (2018). Donepezil, galantamine, rivastigmine and memantine for the treatment of Alzheimer's disease. www.nice.org.uk/guidance/ta217/chapter/1-Guidance.

National Institute for Health and Clinical Excellence (2009). Donepezil, galantamine, rivastigmine (review) and memantine for the treatment of Alzheimer's disease (amended); NICE technology appraisal guidance 111. National Institute for Health and Clinical Excellence: London, UK.

Nordberg, A., Ballard, C., Bullock, R., Darreh-Shori, T., & Somogyi, M. (2013). A review of butyrylcholinesterase as a therapeutic target in the treatment of Alzheimer's disease. *The Primary Care Companion for CNS Disorders*, **15**(2), 26731.

O'Brien, J. T., Holmes, C., Jones, M., et al. (2017). Clinical practice with anti-dementia drugs: A revised (third) consensus statement from the British Association for Psychopharmacology. *Journal of Psychopharmacology*, **31**(2), 147–68.

Rédaction, P. (2018). Médicaments de la maladie d'Alzheimer: Enfin non remboursables en France! *Revue Prescrire*, **38**, 1–2.

Rosen, W. G., Mohs, R. C., & Davis, K. L. (1984). A new rating scale for Alzheimer's disease. *The American Journal of Psychiatry*, **141**, 1356–64. http://dx.doi.org/10.1176/ajp.141.11.1356.

Schneider, L. S., & Qizilbash, N. (2004). Delay in nursing home placement with donepezil. *Journal of the American Geriatric Society*, **52**, 1024–6.

Sims, J. R., Zimmer, J. A., Evans, C. D., et al. (2023). Donanemab in early symptomatic Alzheimer disease: the TRAILBLAZER-ALZ 2 randomized clinical trial. *JAMA*, **330**(6), 512–27.

Therneau, T. M., Knopman, D. S., Lowe, V. J., et al. (2021). Relationships between β-amyloid and tau in an elderly population: An accelerated failure time model. *NeuroImage*, **242**, 118440.

Thomas, S., & Grossberg, G. (2009). Memantine: A review of studies into its safety and efficacy in treating Alzheimer's disease and other dementias. *Clinical Interventions in Aging*, **4**, 367–77.

Walsh, S., Merrick, R., Milne, R. & Brayne, C. (2021). Aducanumab for Alzheimer's disease? *British Medical Journal*, **374**, n1682.

Wessels, A. M., Siemers, E. R., Yu, P., et al. (2015). A combined measure of cognition and function for clinical trials: The integrated Alzheimer's Disease Rating Scale (iADRS). *The Journal of Prevention of Alzheimer's disease*, **2**(4), 227.

World Health Organization (2022). Clinical Trials. www.who.int/health-topics/clinical-trials/#tab=tab_1.

Yang, T., Li, S., Xu, H., Walsh, D. M., Selkoe, D. J. (2017). Large soluble oligomers of amyloid-protein from Alzheimer's brain are far less neuroactive than the smaller oligomers to which they dissociate. *Journal of Neuroscience*, **37**(1), 152–63.

Reducing Risk Factors for Mild Cognitive Impairment and Early Dementia

As the development of pharmacological interventions for mild cognitive impairment (MCI) and dementia has not progressed as rapidly as might have been anticipated, attention has also focussed on non-pharmacological interventions. Although a single cause for most dementias has not been established outside of some of the relatively rare cases linked to specific genes, there are risk factors which increase the likelihood of developing cognitive decline and ultimately dementia. Many of these are covered in Chapter 1, and some are potentially reversible. Livingston et al. (2020) estimated that 12 risk factors could account for up to 40% of all dementias. These were:

- low education levels
- smoking
- excessive alcohol consumption (>21 units per week)
- midlife hypertension
- midlife obesity (BMI>29)
- diabetes
- sedentary lifestyle
- depression
- low social contact
- hearing loss
- traumatic brain injury
- environmental pollution

This chapter will look at some of these factors individually, then consider evidence from programmes which have been established to address a number of these factors by lifestyle changes. It is important to remember that even if it is not possible to completely prevent the development of dementia, delaying onset by 2 years could decrease worldwide prevalence by 22.8 million cases (Brookmeyer et al., 2007).

As with the development of pharmacological interventions, results have not always been consistent, and although evidence for the contribution of certain risk factors leading to cognitive decline may be compelling, addressing those risk factors has not always led to a demonstrable reduction in rates of cognitive decline. One of the reasons for this is likely to be because dementia is multi-factorial, and the resulting cognitive decline probably results from the cumulative effect of all these factors. Therefore, addressing one individual factor may not produce a clinically significant effect. However, combining multiple factors together for an intervention, which is most likely the way forward, raises the question of which factors make a difference. The latter is particularly problematical for setting up randomised control trials, which are considered the gold standard form of evidence.

There are a number of risk factors associated with heart disease, stroke, and cognitive decline. Several programmes have been developed which aim to help people address as many of these risk factors as possible. One of the criticisms of such approaches has been that there are so many lifestyle changes involved, it is unlikely that people will be able to follow all of them (Bredesen, 2017). However, whilst there is stronger evidence for modifying some risk factors than for others, there is no definitive answer as to (1) which ones are most important or (2) whether there is a minimum number which need to be addressed for a programme to be effective. The aim is therefore to assist people to address as many as possible. A key role for psychology is likely to be helping people to stick with the programme, as maintaining a healthy diet and exercise regime is notoriously difficult to achieve (e.g. Moroshko, Brennan, & O-Brien, 2011).

We will first begin by reviewing the interventions for which there is the strongest evidence base. Unfortunately, the literature often indicates that although there may be strong evidence for the role of a particular factor in increasing the risk of developing dementia, this is often not accompanied by equally strong evidence for the effectiveness of reducing that risk factor as a means of preventing dementia. This will be divided into risk factors which can potentially be reduced, and protective factors which can potentially be introduced.

Risk Factors Which May Potentially Be Reduced

Vascular Risk Factors

Vascular risk factors are associated with increased risk of not only vascular but also other common forms of dementia, with up to 80% of Alzheimer's and 61% of frontotemporal dementias having a vascular component (Hachinski et al., 2019). The most common modifiable risk factors for cardiovascular and cerebrovascular disease are high blood pressure, elevated LDL cholesterol, diabetes, and obesity. Atrial fibrillation has also been identified as a major risk factor.

Skoog et al. (1996) conducted a 15-year longitudinal study on a cohort of 70-year-olds, looking at the relationship between blood pressure and the development of dementia. Higher blood pressure at age 70 was associated with the subsequent development of dementia, and an increased number of white matter lesions at age 85. Although there have been numerous trials looking at the effectiveness of anti-hypertensive medication for reducing subsequent rates of dementia in people with high blood pressure, particularly in middle age, results have been inconclusive (Siera, 2020), and a Cochrane review of studies concluded there was no strong evidence for treatment of hypertension reducing subsequent dementia rates (Cunningham et al., 2021).

Cholesterol levels are usually subdivided into HDL (good cholesterol) and LDL (bad cholesterol). In a large study of more than 1.8 million people, Iwagami et al. (2021) reported that there was a 60% higher risk of being diagnosed with dementia after more than 10 years in those whose LDL cholesterol was elevated when measured below the age of 65. The authors stated that this constitutes a bigger risk than alcohol consumption and high blood pressure. The common way of reducing cholesterol levels is by the use of statins. The evidence for the effectiveness of statins in preventing dementia is mixed, although this may partly be due to methodological issues as not all studies have looked for improved cognitive scores in those taking statins when compared to placebo controls. Some studies have reported a protective effect of statins against all forms of dementia (e.g. Wong et al., 2013), but there are also reports of statins causing a decline in cognitive function, which appears to be reversible on discontinuation of the medication. Once statins were restarted, a reduction in cognitive function was once again observed (Wagstaff et al., 2003). It may be that there are two mechanisms at play: one which confers a degree of long-term protection against dementia and one which may cause a more immediate reduction in cognitive function (Shultz, Patten, & Berlau, 2018). This may contribute to some of the apparent contradictions in research results.

Obesity and diabetes often (but not always) co-occur, and both are risk factors for dementia. The identification of diabetes as a risk factor for dementia (particularly vascular dementia) and Alzheimer's disease has been established for decades (Ott et al., 1996). The use of metformin, a medication commonly used for treatment of diabetes, has been linked with a reduced risk of dementia in people with diabetes (Sherrer et al., 2019), and improved cognitive function in non-diabetic patients with MCI (Koenig et al., 2017). Obesity has been associated with a 28% higher risk of developing dementia over a period of at least 15 years (Ma et al., 2020). The evidence tends to point towards obesity in middle age increasing the risk for subsequent dementia (Hassing et al., 2009), rather than obesity in adults over 65 (Dahl et al., 2008).

A relationship between atrial fibrillation and subsequent development of dementia was first suggested in the 1970s, although empirical evidence to support this did not accumulate until sometime later (e.g. Ott et al., 1997). Treatment with oral anticoagulants has been demonstrated in some studies to reduce the subsequent incidence of dementia patients with this condition (e.g. Bezabhe et al., 2022; Friberg & Rosenqvist, 2018).

Tobacco, Alcohol, and Recreational Drugs

In the context of the cholinergic hypothesis of Alzheimer's disease, there have been suggestions that smoking may have a protective effect as nicotine is a substance which stimulates cholinergic receptors. Whilst there is some evidence that smoking may produce short-term improvements in cognitive ability (Kutlu & Gould, 2015), there is considerable evidence that it increases the risk of developing dementia (Zong et al., 2015). There is also evidence that smoking cessation reduces that risk (Choi, Choi, & Park, 2018).

As with tobacco, alcohol has at times been suggested to have some degree of protective function, specifically a dose-dependent one. The relationship between alcohol consumption and dementia risk is often described as 'J-shaped', because low to moderate consumption has either (1) not been shown to increase the risk of developing dementia or (2) been shown to be protective (Peters et al., 2008). There is some uncertainty about what constitutes a safe level of intake in terms of dementia risk, but Weigmann et al. (2020) suggested a cut-off point of around 14 units/week. It is worth noting that although there has been some evidence of possible protective effects of light alcohol use, no programme advocates adding alcohol to your diet.

There has been a lot of recent interest in the medicinal properties of cannabis, and some investigations have been carried out into possible benefits of cannabis for treating some of the psychiatric aspects of dementia (Peprah & McCormack, 2019). Investigations into the effect of recreational cannabis on cognition typically indicate a negative effect (Kroon, Kuhns, & Cousijn, 2021). Meier et al. (2022) reported cognitive deficits and smaller hippocampal volumes in 1,037 individuals followed up from the ages of 18 to 45, which they classified as risks for developing dementia in later life. Whilst clear evidence for cannabis use as a risk factor for the development of dementia appears to be lacking at present, cannabis use may be part of a lifestyle which includes use of other substances such as alcohol, tobacco, and benzodiazepines, the combined use of which may increase risk (Hulse et al., 2005).

Depression

There is an established relationship between depression and dementia, although there is some uncertainty regarding whether depression contributes to the development of dementia or is a prodromal feature (Bennet & Thomas, 2014). A reduction in cognitive function is often a feature of depression, and treatment with anti-depressant medication has been associated with some improvement in cognitive ability, although not necessarily full restoration (Butters et al., 2000). Almeida et al. (2017) completed a 14-year longitudinal study of 4,922 cognitively unimpaired men aged 17–84. They found that the presence of current or past depression was a risk factor for development of future dementia but found no evidence to suggest that anti-depressant medication resulted in risk reduction. Bartels et al. (2018) reported that in non-depressed patients with MCI and a past history of depression, long-term use of SSRIs (>4 years) was associated with an average delay in progression to dementia of 3 years. This effect was not seen with short-term SSRI use or with other forms of anti-depressants.

Whether treatment of depression reduces the risk of subsequent dementia is a question which requires further research. As successful treatment of depression is an end in itself, the issue of the development (or not) of subsequent dementia is unlikely to affect whether treatment is given.

Protective Factors Which May Be Increased

Physical Exercise

The beneficial effects of exercise on physical health have been appreciated for a long time; however, more recently there has been a large increase in research on the possible benefits of exercise on cognition. Ahlskog et al. (2011) carried out a meta-analysis on aerobic exercise and dementia risk, concluding that midlife exercise reduced the risk of subsequently developing dementia or MCI. In studies comparing an exercise group to sedentary controls, increased hippocampal volume was found after 6–12 months of exercise. Resistance training has been considered in several studies, as well as multi-component programmes which combine resistance and aerobic training. Overall, resistance training appears to confer the biggest improvement in global cognition for people with dementia, whereas combined, multi-component exercise is more effective for people with MCI (Huang et al., 2022).

Cognitive Stimulation

A higher level of education has long been recognised as a protective factor against cognitive decline, which is linked with the theory of cognitive reserve (Stern, 2006). Maintaining higher levels of cognitive stimulation with activities such as reading and playing games is also associated with reduced dementia risk (Fratiglioni & Wang, 2007). The English Longitudinal Study of Ageing looked at range of cognitively stimulating activities and reported that internet use and volunteering were associated with a reduced risk of dementia, whereas other activities such as evening classes and paid employment showed no association (Williams, Pendleton, & Chandola, 2020).

Social Engagement

It is well-established that people with dementia have lower levels of social activity, although this may be because cognitive decline leads to less socialising. Some studies have shown that higher levels of leisure activity are associated with a lower risk of developing dementia (Wang et al., 2002), as is having a richer social network (Fratiglioni et al., 2000). Many social activities also involve cognitive stimulation and physical activity (e.g. dance classes, Tai Chi, pursuing outdoor activities), making it unclear which is the most important component. Karp et al. (2006) rated leisure activities according to how much of each component (socialising, cognitive stimulation, physical activity) they involved. They then looked at the levels and types of activity in 776 healthy elderly people over a 6-year period, as a predictor of incident dementia. Their results suggested that all three components reduced the risk of dementia, with the strongest effects for people who engaged in activities with high ratings in at least two of the components.

Healthy Diet

Diets which are high in saturated fat, sugar, and salt, as well as low in fibre, are considered to increase vascular risk. Consequently, a diet which reduces these components is also likely to confer a degree of protection against dementia. Diet can be a difficult area to study, particularly when attempting large-scale studies such as randomised control trials. Consequently, there is a lack of strong evidence for the effectiveness of particular diets for the prevention of dementia, although some evidence is starting to emerge, particularly for the Mediterranean diet and the Keto diet. Morris et al. (2015) followed up 923 participants over 4.5 years on 3 diet protocols: the Mediterranean diet, the Dietary Approaches to Stop Hypertension diet (DASH), and a hybrid of the two (the MIND diet). The hybrid consisted of mainly plant-based foods, with a limited intake of animal products and saturated fat: it also features consumption of berries and green leafy vegetables. While all three diets were associated with lower rates of dementia, the Mediterranean and DASH diets required a high level of adherence to be successful, whereas a modest adherence to the MIND diet still reduced risk.

The ketogenic diet was developed in the 1920s as a treatment for epilepsy (Conklin, 1922), but has gained popularity as a means of weight loss and controlling diabetes (Abbasi, 2018). This is a form of high fat, low carbohydrate diet, but differs from other low carbohydrate diets in that carbohydrate intake is restricted to a far greater extent. Research into the potential of the ketogenic diet is not as advanced as for the other diets mentioned here, but there is some evidence for improved quality of life in adults with Alzheimer's disease, although a significant effect on cognitive scores has yet to be demonstrated (Phillips et al., 2021).

Sleep

Sub-optimal levels of sleep have been associated with a whole range of serious and chronic health conditions, including dementia (Walker, 2017). Sleep fragmentation, or disrupted sleep, is associated with a 1.5-fold increase in the incidence of dementia (Lim et al., 2013).

The optimum amount of sleep per night appears to be 7–8 hours, with both short sleep duration (<7 hours) and long sleep duration (>8 hours) being associated with an increased dementia risk of up to 86% (Bubu et al., 2017).

As yet, there are no studies which have shown that manipulating the amount of sleep per night to 7–8 hours in people previously outside these parameters results in a reduced risk of dementia. However, this may be hard to do in practice, as sleep correction can be difficult to achieve and sustain. Ageing is also associated with a reduced ability to achieve optimum duration and quality of sleep (Mander, Winer, & Walker, 2017).

Dietary Supplements and Medications

A number of dietary supplements have been cited as potentially improving cognitive function, such as ginko biloba, omega-3 fish oils, vitamin E, vitamin B, and curcumin. These are often recommended in complementary health articles and feature in some treatment programmes (e.g. Bredesen, 2017). There are presentations where a deficiency in particular vitamins may lead to cognitive impairment (e.g. vitamin B in Wernicke–Korsakoff's), and supplemental doses may lead to improvement or prevent further damage. The use of vitamins for treatment in this way is backed by strong evidence. The usefulness of supplements for reducing risk of cognitive decline is not currently supported by a strong evidence base (Forbes et al., 2015; Hellmuth, Rabinovici, & Miller, 2019), and there is no evidence to indicate the use of supplements can prevent, treat, or reverse the development of dementia (Helmuth, 2020).

Programmes Combining Multiple Components

A number of programmes aim at reducing the risk of developing dementia by targeting multiple known risk factors. One protocol, ReCODE, designed by Dr Dale Bredesen, has become well-known since the publication of his best-selling book *The End of Alzheimer's* (2017). The protocol includes addressing most of the risk factors described in this chapter, as well as an extensive range of dietary supplements. Whilst Bredesen outlines a coherent rationale for the protocol and makes very strong claims for its effectiveness, the supporting evidence has been strongly criticised (Daly & Mastroleo, 2022; Helmuth, 2020). Evidence cited consists of multiple case studies, rather than controlled trials, and there has been criticism about the depth of information provided in many of the cases.

The Finnish Geriatric Intervention Study to Prevent Cognitive Impairment (FINGER) is an ongoing RCT looking at multi-component strategies to prevent dementia (Ngandu et al., 2015). The initial stages consisted of a two-year intervention period, utilising physical exercise, nutritional guidance, cognitive training, social activity, and management of metabolic and vascular risk factors. The control group received general health advice. The overall risk of developing dementia was 30% higher in the control group. The study is expanding to create a global network of centres following this model (www.alz.org/wwfingers/over view.asp).

Other large-scale trials, such as the French Multi-Domain Alzheimer Preventative trial (MAPT) (Andrieu et al., 2017), which featured lifestyle changes alongside omega-3 fish-oil supplements, and the Dutch Prevention of Dementia by Intensive Vascular Care (PreDIVA) (van Charante et al., 2016), which focussed on pharmacological interventions for vascular risk factors, did not report significant benefits in their primary outcomes.

Key Points

- Whilst there is rarely one clear cause for dementia, there are a number of risk factors which make the development of dementia more likely.
- Many risk factors are potentially reversible. Although addressing all of them may not be possible for many people, reversing some of them may still stop or slow down cognitive decline.
- Risk factors for heart disease and stroke (e.g. high blood pressure, high cholesterol, diabetes, and atrial fibrillation) also increase the risk of developing dementia. These can often be addressed with medical intervention.
- Other risk factors are more successfully address by lifestyle changes.
- Stopping smoking, reducing alcohol consumption, and following a healthy diet are important steps which can be taken.
- Increasing exercise and quantity and quality of sleep are important positive steps which can be taken.
- Although vitamin and dietary supplements are often claimed to improve cognitive ability, evidence for their effectiveness is lacking.
- A number of ongoing research trials are looking at the effect of reducing risk factors, some of which are international and planning to recruit further collaborators.

References

Abbasi, J. Interest in the ketogenic diet grows for weight loss and type 2 diabetes. (2018). *JAMA*, **319**(3), 215–217.

Ahlskog, J. E., Geda, Y. E., Graff-Radford, N. R. and Petersen, R. C. (2011). Physical exercise as a preventive or disease-modifying treatment of dementia and brain aging. *Mayo Clinic Proceedings*, **86**(9), 876–84.

Almeida, O. P., Hankey, G. J., Yeap, B. B., Golledge, J., & Flicker, L. (2017). Depression as a modifiable factor to decrease the risk of dementia. *Translational Psychiatry*, 7(5), e1117–e1117.

Andrieu, S., Guyonnet, S., Coley, N., et al. (2017). Effect of long-term omega 3 polyunsaturated fatty acid supplementation with or without multidomain intervention on cognitive function in elderly adults with memory complaints (MAPT): A randomised, placebo-controlled trial. *The Lancet Neurology*, **16**(5), 377–89.

Bartels, C., Wagner, M., Wolfsgruber, S., et al. (2018). Impact of SSRI therapy on risk of conversion from mild cognitive impairment to Alzheimer's dementia in individuals with previous depression. *American Journal of Psychiatry*, **175**(3), 232–41.

Bennett, S., & Thomas, A. J. (2014). Depression and dementia: Cause, consequence or coincidence?. *Maturitas*, **79**(2), 184–190.

Bezabhe, W. M., Bereznicki, L. R., Radford, J., et al. (2022). Oral anticoagulant treatment and the risk of dementia in patients with atrial fibrillation: A population-based cohort study. *Journal of the American Heart Association*, **11**(7), e023098.

Bredesen, D. (2017). *The End of Alzheimer's Programme: The Practical Plan to Prevent and Reverse Cognitive Decline at Any Age.* London: Vermillion.

Brookmeyer, R., Johnson, E., Ziegler-Graham, K., & Arrighi, H. M. (2007). Forecasting the global burden of Alzheimer's disease. *Alzheimer's & Dementia*, **3**(3), 186–91.

Bubu, O. M., Brannick, M., Mortimer, J., et al. (2017). Sleep, cognitive impairment, and

Alzheimer's disease: A systematic review and meta-analysis. *Sleep*, **40**(1), zsw032.

Butters, M. A., Becker, J. T., Nebes, R. D., et al. (2000). Changes in cognitive functioning following treatment of late-life depression. *American Journal of Psychiatry*, **157**(12), 1949–54.

Choi, D., Choi, S., & Park, S. M. (2018). Effect of smoking cessation on the risk of dementia: A longitudinal study. *Annals of Clinical and Translational Neurology*, **5**(10), 1192–9.

Conklin, H. W. (1922). Cause and treatment of epilepsy. *Journal of the American Osteopathy Association*, **26**, 11–14

Cunningham, E. L., Todd, S. A., Passmore, P., Bullock, R., & McGuinness, B. (2021). Pharmacological treatment of hypertension in people without prior cerebrovascular disease for the prevention of cognitive impairment and dementia. *Cochrane Database of Systematic Reviews*, **5**(5), CD004034. https://doi.org/10.1002/1465185 8.CD004034.pub4.

Dahl, A. K., Löppönen, M., Isoaho, R., Berg, S., & Kivelä, S. L. (2008). Overweight and obesity in old age are not associated with greater dementia risk: *Journal of the American Geriatrics Society*, **56**(12), 2261–6.

Dalya, T., & Mastroleob, I. (2022). The first survivors of Alzheimer's: How patients recovered life and hope in their own words by Dale Bredesen, Avery, 2021, 272 pp. *Journal of Alzheimer's Disease*, **86**, 49–52.

Forbes, S. C., Holroyd-Leduc, J. M., Poulin, M. J., & Hogan, D. B. (2015). Effect of nutrients, dietary supplements and vitamins on cognition: A systematic review and meta-analysis of randomized controlled trials. *Canadian Geriatrics Journal*, **18**(4), 231.

Fratiglioni, L., & Wang, H. X. (2007). Brain reserve hypothesis in dementia. *Journal of Alzheimers Disease*, **12**(1), 11–22.

Fratiglioni, L., Wang, H. X., Ericsson, K., Maytan, M., & Winblad, B. (2000). Influence of social network on occurrence of dementia: a community-based longitudinal study. *Lancet*, **355**, 1315–19.

Friberg, L., & Rosenqvist, M. (2018). Less dementia with oral anticoagulation in atrial fibrillation. *European Heart Journal*, **39**(6), 453–60.

Hachinski, V., Einhäupl, K., Ganten, D., et al. (2019). Preventing dementia by preventing stroke: The Berlin Manifesto. *Alzheimer's & Dementia*, **15**(7), 961–84.

Hassing, L. B., Dahl, A. K., Thorvaldsson, V., et al. (2009). Overweight in midlife and risk of dementia: A 40-year follow-up study. *International Journal of Obesity*, **33**(8), 893–8.

Hellmuth, J. (2020). Can we trust The End of Alzheimer's? *The Lancet. Neurology*, **19** (5), 389.

Hellmuth, J., Rabinovici, G. D., & Miller, B. L. (2019). The rise of pseudomedicine for dementia and brain health. *JAMA*, **321**(6), 543–4.

Huang, X., Zhao, X., Li, B., et al. (2022). Comparative efficacy of various exercise interventions on cognitive function in patients with mild cognitive impairment or dementia: A systematic review and network meta-analysis. *Journal of Sport and Health Science*, **11**, 212–23

Hulse, G. K., Lautenschlager, N. T., Tait, R. J., & Almeida, O. P. (2005). Dementia associated with alcohol and other drug use. *International Psychogeriatrics*, **17**(s1), S109–S127.

Iwagami, M., Qizilbash, N., Gregson, J., et al. (2021). Blood cholesterol and risk of dementia in more than 1.8 million people over two decades: A retrospective cohort study. *The Lancet Healthy Longevity*, **2**(8), e498–e506.

Karp, A., Paillard-Borg, S., Wang, H. X., et al. (2006). Mental, physical and social components in leisure activities equally contribute to decrease dementia risk. *Dementia and Geriatric Cognitive Disorders*, **21**(2), 65–73.

Koenig, A. M., Mechanic-Hamilton, D., Xie, S. X., et al. (2017). Effects of the insulin sensitizer metformin in Alzheimer disease: Pilot data from a randomized placebo-controlled crossover study. *Alzheimer Disease & Associated Disorders*, **31**(2), 107–13.

Kroon, E., Kuhns, L., & Cousijn, J. (2021). The short-term and long-term effects of cannabis on cognition: Recent advances in the field. *Current Opinion in Psychology*, **38**, 49–55.

Kutlu, M. G., & Gould, T. J. (2015). Nicotinic receptors, memory, and hippocampus. *The Neurobiology and Genetics of Nicotine and Tobacco*, **23**, 137–63.

Lim, A. S., Kowgier, M., Yu, L., Buchman, A. S., & Bennett, D. A. (2013). Sleep fragmentation and the risk of incident Alzheimer's disease and cognitive decline in older persons. *Sleep*, **36**(7), 1027–32.

Livingston, G., Huntley, J., Sommerlad, A., et al. (2020). Dementia prevention, intervention, and care: 2020 report of the Lancet Commission. *The Lancet*, **396**(10248), 413–46.

Ma, Y., Ajnakina, O., Steptoe, A., & Cadar, D. (2020). Higher risk of dementia in English older individuals who are overweight or obese. *International Journal of Epidemiology*, **49**(4), 1353–65.

Mander, B. A., Winer, J. R., & Walker, M. P. (2017). Sleep and human aging. *Neuron*, **94**(1), 19–36.

Meier, M. H., Caspi, A. R., Knodt, A., et al. (2022). Long-term cannabis use and cognitive reserves and hippocampal volume in midlife. *American Journal of Psychiatry*, **179**(5), 362–74.

Moroshko, I., Brennan, L., & O'Brien, P. (2011). Predictors of dropout in weight loss interventions: A systematic review of the literature. *Obesity Reviews*, **12**(11), 912–34.

Morris, M. C., Tangney, C. C., Wang, Y., et al. (2015). MIND diet associated with reduced incidence of Alzheimer's disease. *Alzheimer's & Dementia*, **11**(9), 1007–14.

Ngandu, T., Lehtisalo, J., Solomon, A., et al. (2015). A 2 year multidomain intervention of diet, exercise, cognitive training, and vascular risk monitoring versus control to prevent cognitive decline in at-risk elderly people (FINGER): A randomised controlled trial. *The Lancet*, **385**(9984), 2255–63.

Ott, A., Breteler, M. M., De Bruyne, M. C., et al. (1997). Atrial fibrillation and dementia in a population-based study: The Rotterdam Study. *Stroke*, **28**(2), 316–21.

Ott, A., Stolk, R. P., Hofman, A., et al. (1996). Association of diabetes mellitus and dementia: The Rotterdam Study. *Diabetologia*, **39**, 1392–7.

Peprah, K., & McCormack, S. (2019). Medical cannabis for the treatment of dementia: a review of clinical effectiveness and guidelines. Review from Canadian Agency for Drugs and Technologies in Health, Ottawa (ON). www.ncbi.nlm.nih.gov/books/NBK546328/.

Peters, R., Peters, J., Warner, J., Beckett, N., & Bulpitt, C. (2008). Alcohol, dementia and cognitive decline in the elderly: A systematic review. *Age and Ageing*, **37**(5), 505–12.

Phillips, M. C., Deprez, L. M., Mortimer, G., et al. (2021). Randomized crossover trial of a modified ketogenic diet in Alzheimer's disease. *Alzheimer's Research & Therapy*, **13**(1), 1–12.

Scherrer, J. F., Morley, J. E., Salas, J., et al. (2019). Association between metformin initiation and incident dementia among African American and white veterans' health administration patients. *The Annals of Family Medicine*, **17**(4), 352–62.

Schultz, B. G., Patten, D. K., & Berlau, D. J. (2018). The role of statins in both cognitive impairment and protection against dementia: A tale of two mechanisms. *Translational Neurodegeneration*, **7**, 1–11.

Sierra, C. (2020). Hypertension and the risk of dementia. *Frontiers in Cardiovascular Medicine*, **7**, 5.

Skoog, I., Nilsson, L., Persson, G., et al. (1996). 15-year longitudinal study of blood pressure and dementia. *The Lancet*, **347**(9009), 1141–5.

Stern, Y. (2006). Cognitive reserve and Alzheimer disease. *Alzheimer Disease and Associated Disorders*, **20**(3)(**suppl 2**), S69–S74.

van Charante, E. P. M., Richard, E., Eurelings, L. S., et al. (2016). Effectiveness of a 6-year multidomain vascular care intervention to prevent dementia (preDIVA): A cluster-randomised controlled trial. *The Lancet*, **388**(10046), 797–805.

Wagstaff, L., Mitton, M., Arvik, B., & Doraiswamy, P. (2003). Statin-associated memory loss: Analysis of 60 case reports and review of the literature. *Pharmacotherapy*, **23**, 871–80.

Walker, M. (2017). *Why We Sleep*. Allen Lane.

Wang, H. X., Karp, A., Winblad, B., & Fratiglioni, L. (2002). Late-life engagement in social and leisure activities is associated with a decreased risk of dementia: A longitudinal study from the Kungsholmen Project. *American Journal of Epidemiology*, **155**, 1081–7.

Wiegmann, C., Mick, I., Brandl, E. J., Heinz, A., & Gutwinski, S. (2020). Alcohol and dementia – what is the link? A systematic review. *Neuropsychiatric Disease and Treatment*, **16** 87–99.

Williams, B. D., Pendleton, N., & Chandola, T. (2020). Cognitively stimulating activities and risk of probable dementia or cognitive impairment in the English Longitudinal Study of Ageing. *SSM – Population Health*, **12**, 100656.

Wong, W. B., Lin, V. W., Boudreau, D., & Devine, E. B. (2013). Statins in the prevention of dementia and Alzheimer's disease: A meta-analysis of observational studies and an assessment of confounding. *Pharmacoepidemiology and Drug Safety*, **22**(4), 345–58.

Zhong, G., Wang, Y., Zhang, Y., Guo, J. J., & Zhao, Y. (2015). Smoking is associated with an increased risk of dementia: A meta-analysis of prospective cohort studies with investigation of potential effect modifiers. *PloS One*, **10**(3), e0118333.

Biomarkers and Imaging

There have been various definitions of what constitutes a biological maker (biomarker). For the purposes of this chapter, we will use a definition put forward in 1998 by the National Institutes of Health Biomarkers Definitions Working Group of 'a characteristic that is objectively measured and evaluated as an indicator of normal biological processes, pathogenic processes, or pharmacologic responses to a therapeutic intervention' (Biomarkers Working Definitions Working Group, 2001). An *imaging biomarker* is one that is detectable in an image (Smith, Sorensen, & Thrall, 2003). This chapter will consider the use of biomarkers in the diagnosis of dementia, covering imaging biomarkers and progressing through to fluid biomarkers. Whilst the use of biomarkers has become an essential component of research into dementia and mild cognitive impairment, the use of such technologies (other than structural imaging) has yet to become widely incorporated into clinical practice, and this may remain the case for some years. Diagnosis of dementia is still firmly based on clinical history, cognitive ability, and everyday function (e.g. DSM-V, ICD-11), but biomarkers are likely to play an increasingly important role in classification of dementia subtype and underlying pathology.

It is important to note that interpretation of scans and other biological investigations requires training, and when a scan is interpreted a report is produced. It is, however, important for non-radiologists to have sufficient background knowledge to integrate the scan report with the other sources of information which lead to a diagnosis.

Structural Imaging: Computerised Tomography (CT) and Magnetic Resonance Imagery (MRI)

CT and MRI scans produce internal images of the body. Although the initial purpose of CT scans was to exclude non-dementia causes for cognitive decline, such as tumours, they have become increasingly important for identifying (1) generalised and localised patterns of brain atrophy and (2) areas of ischaemic change. The images can be viewed as a series of slices through the brain from front to back (coronal), bottom to top (axial), and side to side (sagittal).

CT scans work by taking a series of X-ray images. MRI uses a powerful magnet which aligns the body's water molecules. A radio frequency is then passed through the tissue, which puts the water molecules out of alignment. As they realign, signals are sent to receivers which create a detailed image because different tissue types realign at different speeds.

Atrophy is the medical term for shrinkage. Degenerative and cerebrovascular disorders are associated with a reduction in the overall size of the brain (generalised atrophy) and/or a relative reduction in size of specific brain regions (e.g. the medial temporal lobe in Alzheimer's disease). CT and MRI scans can both detect atrophy, which shows as an increase in the amount of space inside the skull, and an increase in the size of the gaps (sulci) between the folds (gyri) of the cortex. Although MRI produces higher-resolution images and is considered to be the preferred imaging technique for dementia diagnosis (Harper et al., 2014), it is not always the most readily available. There is also a lack of clear evidence that use of MRI over CT delivers greater accuracy in distinguishing vascular dementia from Alzheimer's, or mixed dementia (Benyon et al., 2012). The London Dementia Clinical Network (Orleans-Foli, Isaacs, & Cook, 2018) advocates the use of CT over MRI, unless dementia subtype is undecided and vascular dementia is a consideration. These authors argue against the routine use of scans in dementia diagnosis for all patients, pointing out that (1) the majority of patients under 60 referred to memory assessment services do not have dementia, and (2) imaging may not be informative in patients over the age of 80 as neuroradiological changes are less specific and overlap more with regular ageing.

Harper et al. (2014) outlined 'an algorithmic approach to structural imaging in dementia', which has been widely adopted for evaluating patterns of atrophy and ischaemic damage considered indicative of the underlying causes of dementia and MCI. Although primarily intended for MRI, they acknowledge that 'CT can be used relatively effectively to evaluate the presence and extent of cerebrovascular disease' (p. 693). This approach consists of several indices of atrophy, graded for severity:

- GTA: a global cortical atrophy scale ranging from 0 (no atrophy) to 3 (severe) (Pasquier et al., 1996).
- MTA: a medial temporal lobe atrophy score (Sheltens et al., 1992), which is considered particularly important for identifying Alzheimer's disease. The scores range from 0 (no atrophy) to 4 (severe loss of volume in the hippocampal region). A score of 2 or more is considered abnormal for individuals under the age of 75, with a score of 3 or more being abnormal for those aged 75 and over.
- The Koedam score assesses parietal lobe atrophy and is scored from 0 to 3. (Koedam et al., 2011).

Ischaemic change is rated according to two indices:

- The Fazekas scale for the number of white matter lesions, graded from 0 to 3 (Wahlund et al., 2001).
- Strategic infarcts, which are sites of ischaemic damage in crucial areas for normal cognition.

Sample images of different levels atrophy and ischaemia according to these indices can be found online via sites such as Radiology Assistant (see, e.g. https://radiologyassistant.nl/neuroradiology/dementia/role-of-mri).

Harper et al. (2014) summarise several patterns which are characteristic of particular disorders, although often not exclusively so. They also point out that when no abnormalities are detected and a scan is reported as 'within normal limits', this does not rule out dementia or degenerative processes. A summary of characteristics associated with particular degenerative forms of dementia is shown in Table 13.1.

At present, most CT/MRI scan interpretation involves a visual inspection of scan images; however, a more automated alternative of volumetric analysis has also been developed, which could potentially increase diagnostic accuracy (Pemberton et al., 2021). This has yet to be incorporated into widespread clinical practice.

Table 13.1 Patterns of atrophy associated with cause of dementia, adapted from Harper et al. (2014)

Pattern seen	Associated pathology
Generalised atrophy	A non-specific finding associated with Alzheimer's disease, Lewy body dementia, and vascular disease. Can also be seen with normal ageing
Medial temporal lobe (hippocampal) atrophy	Alzheimer's disease. Can be used to distinguish AD from DLB, as this is absent from DLB in the early stages. Also seen in hippocampal sclerosis
Asymmetrical temporal lobe atrophy	Can be associated with AD, but more commonly with FTD. Semantic dementia is characterised by pronounced left temporal lobe atrophy, whereas right-sided more commonly presents as behavioural variant (sometimes with prosopagnosia)
Disproportionate frontal lobe atrophy	Behavioural variant FTD (can be symmetrical or asymmetrical)
Parietal/occipital lobe atrophy	Posterior cortical atrophy

Functional Imaging: Single-Photon Emission Computed Tomography (SPECT) and Positron Emission Tomography (PET)

SPECT and PET are methods of functional imaging which have been used in dementia research and are becoming more common in clinical practice. Instead of looking at brain structure, these types of imaging focus on metabolism. Both techniques can be used to detect changes in cerebral blood flow, which can be evident before structural changes are apparent (Vallotassiou et al., 2011). SPECT and PET both make use of injecting radioactive tracers but differ in the type of tracer used and the equipment required. PET uses a positron emitting radioisotope, whereas SPECT uses isotopes which emit gamma rays (Radiopedia, 2023). SPECT has less sensitivity and specificity for differential diagnosis than PET (O'Brien et al., 2014), but costs less and is consequently more widely available in clinical practice. One of the common uses of SPECT is a DaTscan: this looks at dopamine reuptake in the basal ganglia, which is reduced in Parkinson's disease (McKeith et al., 2017; also see Chapter 7). The ability to detect this allows a DaTscan to be used in the diagnosis of Parkinson's disease, to dementia with Lewy bodies (DLB), Parkinsonian disorders, and differentiation of these from Alzheimer's disease (Yeo et al., 2013).

PET scans have been demonstrated to be superior to SPECT in distinguishing between patients with dementia and healthy controls, as well as between those with Alzheimer's and Lewy body dementia (O'Brien et al., 2014). FDG-PET (^{18}F-fluorodeoxyglucose-positron emission tomography) measures brain metabolism via the uptake of glucose in different brain regions. Reduced uptake in the temporo-parietal regions and the posterior cingulate cortex is associated with Alzheimer's disease, and amnestic MCI with progression to Alzheimer's dementia (Anchisi et al., 2005). Whilst FGD-PET has been reported to be highly successful at distinguishing patients with AD from healthy controls, it is less useful for distinguishing Alzheimer's dementia from MCI or other forms of dementia (Bloudek et al., 2011).

Amyloid PET scans use a different type of tracer to an FDG-PET, which can measure the uptake by beta amyloid protein and can therefore indicate its density and distribution. This technology is being utilised extensively in drug trials, particularly those aimed at clearing or reducing amyloid load (Khoury & Ghossoub, 2019). Amyloid PET scans are likely to become increasingly important as drug trials move more into preclinical stages, as they can determine whether amnestic MCI is due to underlying Alzheimer pathology (Albert et al., 2011). Tracers have also been developed for tau protein, which is more closely associated with structural changes and cognitive decline than beta amyloid (Hanseeuw et al., 2019).

Fluid Biomarkers

Extraction and analysis of cerebrospinal fluid (CFS) by lumbar puncture is a diagnostic tool that has been commonly used by neurologists for many years, particularly in the diagnosis of multiple sclerosis (Poser & Brinar, 2001). More recently, this technique has been used to identity the presence of abnormal beta amyloid protein. In the early stages of Alzheimer's disease, CFS amyloid can be detected before it shows on an amyloid PET scan, and before structural changes can be detected on CT or MRI (Palmqvist, Matteson, & Hansson, 2016). CFS tau levels can also be informative, as total CFS tau level can be associated with a range of different pathologies, but particularly frontotemporal dementia (FTD) (Lewczuk et al., 2018).

Less invasive means of investigation, such as blood and saliva analysis, have also been considered, but more research is required to establish the utility of these options.

Biomarkers in Clinical Practice

Although the use of biomarkers has become the gold standard for research, there is always a delay before new developments become incorporated into routine clinical practice. There are challenges with PET and CFS analysis in that PET is expensive and not widely available, and CFS analysis is a relatively invasive procedure. However, with the development of new drugs to remove abnormal proteins before dementia develops, a reliable method of identifying diseases such as Alzheimer's at preclinical stages will be essential. It has been reported that up to 25% of patients diagnosed with mild Alzheimer's and up to 50% of patients with a diagnosis of MCI are subsequently not found to have evidence of beta amyloid deposits (Khoury & Ghossoub, 2019), and therefore would gain no benefits from amyloid-reducing medications.

It should also be noted that beta amyloid protein accumulates with age and is found in the brains of cognitively intact older adults. Mixed presentations are also relatively common in older adults (e.g. over 80 years of age), so the detection of beta amyloid may be an incidental finding. The use of biomarkers is therefore more likely to be of high importance in the early stages of a progressive illness, and in those who are unlikely to have multiple pathologies.

Key Points

- Although diagnosis of dementia is based on clinical presentation, biomarkers have become increasingly important in the differential diagnosis of dementia subtypes.
- Imaging biomarkers include CT and MRI scans, which look at brain structure, and functional imaging such as SPECT and PET, which look at patterns of brain activity.
- Amyloid PET scans have been widely incorporated into research protocols and are able to determine whether patients with amnestic MRI do in fact have a preclinical stage of Alzheimer's disease. However, PET scans are relatively expensive and not widely available.
- CFS analysis is also able to identify a build-up of beta amyloid, sometimes before it is detectable by PET scan and before structural changes are evident. Whilst cheaper than a PET scan, CFS analysis requires a lumbar puncture, which is a relatively invasive procedure.
- A purely biological diagnostic system has been proposed for Alzheimer's disease. However, this is unlikely to be used in clinical practice for some time.

References

Albert, M. S., DeKosky, S. T., Dickson, D., et al. (2011). The diagnosis of mild cognitive impairment due to Alzheimer's disease: Recommendations from the National Institute on Aging-Alzheimer's Association workgroups on diagnostic guidelines for Alzheimer's disease. *Alzheimer's & Dementia: The Journal of the Alzheimer's Association*, 7(3), 270–9.

Anchisi, D., Borroni, B., Franceschi, M., et al. (2005). Heterogeneity of brain glucose metabolism in mild cognitive impairment and clinical progression to Alzheimer disease. *Archives of Neurology*, 62(11), 1728–33.

Beynon, R., Sterne, J. A., Wilcock, G., et al. (2012). Is MRI better than CT for detecting a vascular component to dementia? A systematic review and meta-analysis. *BMC Neurology*, 12(1), 1–10.

Biomarkers Working Definitions Group (2001). Biomarkers and surrogate endpoints: preferred definitions and conceptual framework. *Clinical Pharmacology and Therapeutics*, 69(3), 89–96.

Bloudek, L. M., Spackman, D. E., Blankenburg, M., & Sullivan, S. D. (2011). Review and meta-analysis of biomarkers and diagnostic imaging in Alzheimer's disease. *Journal of Alzheimer's Disease*, 26(4), 627–45.

Hanseeuw, B. J., Betensky, R. A., Jacobs, H. I., et al. (2019). Association of amyloid and tau with cognition in preclinical Alzheimer disease: A longitudinal study. *JAMA Neurology*, 76(8), 915–24.

Harper, L., Barkhof, F., Scheltens, P., Schott, J. M., & Fox, N. C. (2014). An algorithmic approach to structural imaging in dementia. *Journal of Neurology, Neurosurgery & Psychiatry*, 85(6), 692–8.

Jack Jr, C. R., Bennett, D. A., Blennow, K., et al. (2018). NIA-AA research framework: Toward a biological definition of Alzheimer's disease. *Alzheimer's & Dementia*, 14(4), 535–62.

Khoury, R., & Ghossoub, E. (2019). Diagnostic biomarkers of Alzheimer's disease: A state-of-the-art review. *Biomarkers in Neuropsychiatry*, 1, 100005.

Koedam, E. L., Lehmann, M., van der Flier, W. M., et al. (2011). Visual assessment of posterior atrophy development of a MRI rating scale. *European Radiology*, **21**, 2618–25.

Lewczuk, P., Riederer, P., O'Bryant, S. E., et al. (2018). Cerebrospinal fluid and blood biomarkers for neurodegenerative dementias: An update of the Consensus of the Task Force on Biological Markers in Psychiatry of the World Federation of Societies of Biological Psychiatry. *The World Journal of Biological Psychiatry*, **19**(4), 244–328.

McKeith, I. G., Boeve, B. F., Dickson, D. W., et al. (2017). Diagnosis and management of dementia with Lewy bodies: Fourth consensus report of the DLB Consortium. *Neurology*, **89**(1), 88–100.

O'Brien, J. T., Firbank, M. J., Davison, C., et al. (2014). 18F-FDG PET and perfusion SPECT in the diagnosis of Alzheimer and Lewy body dementias. *Journal of Nuclear Medicine*, **55**(12), 1959–65.

Orleans-Foli, S., Isaacs, S., & Cook, L. (2018). London Dementia Clinical Network Neuroimaging for dementia diagnosis: Guidance from the London Dementia Clinical Network. www.england.nhs.uk/london/wp-content/uploads/sites/8/2019/09/Neuroimaging-for-dementia-diagnosis-London-Dementia-Clinical-Network.pdf.

Palmqvist, S., Mattsson, N., Hansson, O., & Alzheimer's Disease Neuroimaging Initiative. (2016). Cerebrospinal fluid analysis detects cerebral amyloid-β accumulation earlier than positron emission tomography. *Brain*, **139**(4), 1226–36.

Pasquier, F., Leys, D., Weerts, J. G., Mounier-Vehier, F., Barkhof, F., & Scheltens, P. (1996). Inter- and intraobserver reproducibility of cerebral atrophy assessment on MRI scans with hemispheric infarcts. *European Neurology*, **36**(5), 268–72.

Pemberton, H. G., Zaki, L. A., Goodkin, O., et al. (2021). Technical and clinical validation of commercial automated volumetric MRI tools for dementia diagnosis – a systematic review. *Neuroradiology*, **63**(11), 1773–89.

Poser, C. M., & Brinar, V. V. (2001). Diagnostic criteria for multiple sclerosis. *Clinical Neurology and Neurosurgery*, **103**(1), 1–11.

Radiology Assistant. https://radiologyassistant.nl/neuroradiology/dementia/role-of-mri.

Radiopedia (2023). SPECT vs PET. https://radiopaedia.org/articles/spect-vs-pet?lang=gb.

Scheltens, P., Leys, D., Barkhof, F., et al. (1992). Atrophy of medial temporal lobes on MRI in 'probable' Alzheimer's disease and normal ageing: Diagnostic value and neuropsychological correlates. *Journal of Neurology, Neurosurgery & Psychiatry*, **55**(10), 967–72.

Smith, J. J., Sorensen, A. G., & Thrall, J. H. (2003). Biomarkers in imaging: Realizing radiology's future. *Radiology*, **227**(3), 633–8.

Valotassiou, V., Sifakis, N., Paptriantafyllou, J., Angelidis, G., & Georgoulias, P. (2011). The clinical use of SPECT and PET molecular imaging in Alzheimer's disease. In De La Monte, S. (Ed). *The Clinical Spectrum of Alzheimer's Disease*. InTech Open.

Wahlund, L. O., Barkhof, F., Fazekas, F., et al. (2001). A new rating scale for age-related white matter changes applicable to MRI and CT. *Stroke*, **32**(6), 1318–22.

Yeo, J. M., Lim, X., Khan, Z., & Pal, S. (2013). Systematic review of the diagnostic utility of SPECT imaging in dementia. *European Archives of Psychiatry and Clinical Neuroscience*, **263**, 539–52.

14

Dementia and Mental Capacity

What Is the Mental Capacity Act (2005)?

Mental capacity is the ability to understand a situation and make decisions. Although there has always been common law to refer to, the Mental Capacity Act (2005) (MCA) (Department for Constitutional Affairs, 2017) was the first time a set of legislatures was developed specifically to address what to do in cases where people are unable to make their own decisions. Perhaps even more importantly, it introduced a formal method for the assessment of mental capacity rather than relying on anything vaguer. It is important to remember that mental capacity is a legal concept, rather than a medical or psychological one, which means that legal professionals may have considerably more expertise in this area than clinicians and citing relevant case law is often required in a report rather than academic research. Unlike scientific research, application/interpretation of the law can change suddenly following a single relevant court decision.

This has implications for how quickly textbooks and articles can become out dated, including the information in this chapter. An amendment to the act was published in 2019, introducing the concept of Liberty Protection Safeguards, which is due to replace the existing Deprivation of Liberty Safeguards. An updated version of the act was due to be introduced in 2023. At the time of writing, a draft version was available which may still differ from the final version in some ways.

The MCA applies to England and Wales. Scotland, Northern Ireland, and countries outside of the UK have their own legal frameworks which apply specifically to their legal systems. Whilst there may be differences in the details and applications of these different acts, the core principles are likely to be similar.

Whilst a lot of the information contained within this chapter is taken directly from the MCA Code of Conduct, which is a considerably more extensive document, here an attempt is made to highlight the key points which are essential to understand for clinicians working in the field of dementia. The historical development of the MCA along with key cases (e.g. the Bournewood case: *R. v Bournewood Community and Mental Health NHS Trust Ex p. L* [1998] UKHL 24) are extensively documented in many texts and will not be covered here.

Key Points to Understand

Although everyone working within healthcare or social services will have undertaken some basic training in the MCA, confusions can arise that potentially lead to inappropriate requests for assessment. Misunderstandings around the following points have all been frequently encountered by the author in routine clinical practice, and anybody undertaking capacity assessments needs to be aware of these.

1. Mental capacity is always decision specific. It is not possible to make a general statement regarding whether a person has capacity 'in general', although I have received frequent requests to make such pronouncements and indeed have encountered them in reports written by other clinicians. A person may have capacity to make one decision, but that does not mean they do/do not have capacity to make a different decision.

2. Mental capacity is always time specific. The severity of a dysfunction of mind or brain often varies across different time periods. For example, an individual with a mental health problem such as depression may demonstrate fluctuating capacity according to variations in their mood. An individual with an acquired brain injury may lack capacity for a specific decision in the early stages of recovery from their injury and cognitive abilities can show considerable improvement in the acute and post-acute stages of recovery. Conversely, an individual with a progressive degenerative condition such as dementia may retain capacity for a decision during the early stages of their illness but lose capacity as the severity of their cognitive deficits increase. The focus must always be on whether the person has capacity at the time the decision needs to be made. It is not possible to assess capacity retrospectively.

3. Mental capacity and vulnerability may be inter-related, but they are not the same thing. Someone who lacks capacity for a decision may indeed be highly vulnerable to outside influences, but being vulnerable is not a reason to conclude someone lacks capacity. If the person can be shown to lack capacity, the issue would be dealt with via the same legal means as any other issue related to capacity, which in England and Wales is the Court of Protection. However, if a person is vulnerable and cannot be shown to lack capacity, separate legislation exists, known as Inherent Jurisdiction, which is administered by the High Court and may be a more appropriate legal framework.

In the early years following the introduction of the MCA, misunderstanding around the first two points was common; this is less so now. Confusion around the third point appears to persist.

Who Should Undertake Capacity Assessments?

The straightforward answer to this question is anybody with a healthcare, medical, or social work qualification who has undertaken appropriate training. Such assessments should never be undertaken by anybody without an appropriate qualification, even if they are experienced at working with a particular clinical population. Assistant psychologists should not undertake such assessments as their psychology degree is not a professional qualification. The situation with trainees is perhaps less clear as this is a training post, with the trainee undertaking an assessment under close supervision which will be signed off by the qualified supervisor. All clinical work undertaken by trainee clinical psychologists is done under supervision; the supervisor has responsibility for the trainee's clinical work, and will counter-sign any documentation produced by the trainee.

The Five Principles of the MCA

1. Presumption of capacity. This is always the starting point. To rebut that presumption, a case must be made to demonstrate why the person now lacks capacity. Although the term 'assumption' was originally used, it has been suggested that 'presumption' is more

appropriate as this implies something is taken to be true 'on the balance of probabilities' and allows this phrase to be used when summarising conclusions (Farmer, 2017).

2. Supported decision-making should be evidenced when required. All attempts must be made to support the person during assessment, including strategies such as using communication and memory aids, and this must be evidenced in reports or formal documentation of the assessment.

3. Decision-making ability is the key thing to assess, and not the wisdom of the specific decision. We are all capable of making a bad decision even if we have capacity. In practice these concepts may be inter-related, but they must be kept separate for the purposes of a mental capacity assessment.

4. Best interests. If the person is considered to lack capacity, there is a requirement to act in their best interests. This may often require a formal, documented best-interest meeting with all concerned parties present.

5. Least restrictive options. When acting in a person's best interests, least restrictive options should be followed.

Points 1–3 apply in all cases; points 4 and 5 only apply if the person has been demonstrated to lack capacity.

Decisions Covered by the MCA

Although the act can apply to most decisions, the common questions likely to arise in the context of dementia are capacity to:

1. Decide on care and residence
2. Consent to treatment
3. Manage finances
4. Make a will
5. Grant Power of Attorney

A sometimes overlooked question in relation to dementia may also be whether the person has capacity to consent to a dementia assessment.

These points will be covered in more detail later in the chapter.

What Is Not Covered?

As mentioned, most decisions are covered, and you may be asked to carry out an assessment of virtually anything. However, certain decisions are excluded, meaning that any assessment made cannot then be followed up via a best-interest meeting. They are covered by common law and case law, but if someone lacks capacity in relation these decisions they will probably need to be referred to the Court of Protection. Examples of decisions not covered by the MCA are:

- Matters relating to relationships: marriage and civil partnership, divorce and sexual relationships (usually comes under the Sex Offenders Act, 2003)
- Matters relating to parenting: placing a child up for adoption, taking over parental responsibility for a child, fertility treatment
- Legal matters: voting and detention under the Mental Health Act (MHA) (1983)

People Under 18 Years of Age

Although this will not be relevant to most patients referred to a memory clinic, there are dementias which occur predominantly in childhood. It is therefore possible that the question of capacity is raised with such patients. In general, the MCA does not apply to people under the age of 16 as they are covered by the Children's Act (2004). This act does not have its own test of mental capacity, therefore the test from the MCA is still likely to be used. For people aged 16–17, the MCA generally does apply, with three exceptions: granting lasting power of attorney, making a will, and advanced decisions to refuse treatment can only be done by persons over the age of 18.

The Two-Stage Test of Mental Capacity, and the Causative Nexus

The MCA outlines a two-stage test of mental capacity, although it is perhaps more useful to think of it as having three components which must be satisfied:

1. The diagnostic test. For the MCA to apply, there must be evidence for a dysfunction of mind or brain.
2. The functional test. This normally takes the form of one or more interviews, during which the person is given the opportunity to demonstrate whether they can understand, retain, and evaluate information relevant to the specific decision, and to communicate their decision.
3. The causative nexus: if it has been established that the person meets the criteria for the diagnostic test and does not have capacity to make the decision on the basis of the functional test, it must also be clear that the impairment in mind or brain is the reason the person did not pass the functional test.

In the original MCA Code of Practice, the diagnostic test was usually undertaken before the functional test. In the revised version of the act, this order has been reversed (MCA Code of Conduct (draft)).

Setting the Thresholds

Although the MCA Code of Practice sets out the two-stage test, it is down to the individual assessor to decide what is a sufficient threshold for understanding. Farmer (2017) recommends considering the understanding required for any decision in terms of four criteria (CMSL): the Concept is the basic idea behind the decision, the Mechanics are the practicalities involved, the Short-term refers to the immediate implications, and the Long-term refers to the lasting implications. In terms of where to set the threshold of understanding, the 'average man on the street'/'man on the Clapham omnibus' test is recommended, which means what you would expect the 'average' person to know. The person being assessed needs to grasp the salient details, rather than the minute details.

The threshold for retention of information is that the person can retain it for a sufficient period of time to make the decision. Following principle 2 of the MCA, it is acceptable to use whatever support is necessary to assist the person to retain that information, which can include the use of notes and other forms of memory aid. It should be taken into consideration that different decisions will require retention of information over different time periods; for example, capacity to engage in litigation would require relevant information to be retained throughout the entire litigation period, although this may still be achieved with the use of memory aids.

The threshold for communication of a decision is often based upon the extent to which communication can be facilitated. Speech and language therapists are often called upon to assist in this regard.

The threshold for evaluating a decision is related to whether it is possible to demonstrate a degree of reasoning that has led to the conclusion. Techniques such as going through a cost–benefit analysis of the possible outcomes of the decision can be useful in this regard.

Should the Capacity Assessment Include Some Cognitive Testing?

Essentially, the more evidence you have, the stronger your assessment. However, this should be weighed against the person's ability to tolerate assessment, which may be a significant limiting factor. In the case of dementia, which can affect people differently, it will always be useful to understand which aspects of cognition are impaired. In most instances, some form of cognitive assessment will have been undertaken as part of the diagnostic process; however, this may not be considered sufficient or may not have been carried out within a reasonable timescale of the assessment.

Ordinary Power of Attorney, Lasting Power of Attorney, and Court-Appointed Deputies

Power of attorney (POA) is a means whereby someone can appoint another person to make decisions on their behalf. This can be in relation to finances or to health and well-being; these can be granted separately, or the same person may be appointed to cover both. Although these roles overlap, there are some important differences in relation to mental capacity, which are summarised here:

1. OPA is granted by someone who has capacity and applies so long as they still have capacity. Whilst another person is authorised to make decisions on their behalf, the person can overrule these decisions should they not agree. If the person loses capacity, OPA no longer applies.

2. LPA is when someone with capacity grants POA to someone in anticipation of the possible loss of capacity. It must be granted while the person has capacity but does not come into force until such a time as they lose capacity. It also no longer applies should the person regain capacity.

3. If someone lacks capacity and has not appointed a person for LPA, an application to the Court of Protection may be made to appoint someone. This is usually a family member, or sometimes a legal professional. If this person has been appointed by the court rather than having LPA granted to them by the individual, this is known as a court-appointed deputy. There are some differences between LPA and a court-appointed deputy, but both give the right to make decisions on the person's behalf.

Independent Mental Capacity Advocate

The Independent Mental Capacity Advocate (IMCA) is an independent advocate who is instructed to provide support to a person who lacks capacity to make decisions about serious medical treatment and long-term accommodation. They would normally be appointed if there are no suitable family or friends to consult in relation to the person's best interests. They can only act once appointed by the appropriate body, which will be the NHS in relation to medical treatment or the local authority in relation to long-term accommodation.

Fluctuating Capacity

It is possible for a person's capacity for a particular decision to fluctuate. This may be in relation to something directly affecting their cognition, or may possibly represent the effect of changes in mental health. In general, it is thought best to assess the person on multiple occasions when their capacity is likely to be at its best. This applies for a single decision which is likely to be required once (e.g. choice of accommodation or care package). However, some decisions will need to be made on multiple occasions (e.g. whether to accept a particular aspect of treatment which is required regularly). In such cases it is probably necessary to perform some form of capacity assessment every time the need for treatment arises. If the person is likely to regain capacity (e.g. if they are experiencing delirium), it is best to postpone the assessment (where possible) until such time as they are likely to have recovered.

Some Issues to Consider When Considering Capacity and Dementia: The Frontal Lobe Paradox

Before going on to discuss the other major aspect of the MCA, which is deprivation of liberty and the Liberty Protection Safeguards, it is worth pausing to reflect on some issues which are pertinent to dementia. The first thing to consider is how decisions are made, for which I am going to use an analogy put forward by social psychology professor Jonathan Haidt (Haidt, 2006, 2012) of the elephant and the rider. The majority of the human mind functions automatically, but there is a small component which represents conscious, logical thought. When we make a decision, it is mostly an automatic process. When we wish to consider things in more detail, the conscious part comes into play and may exert some control over the automatic part, which is larger and stronger. But if the automatic part is steering strongly in a particular direction, it is questionable how much influence the conscious part may exert. Haidt drew the analogy of a strong, powerful elephant, and a small rider sat on top attempting to influence the direction of travel. If the elephant decides it is going in a particular direction, the rider will find it very difficult to influence the elephant to do otherwise. Although this analogy was not intended to directly describe the relationship between the executive system and the rest of the human brain, it can be a useful way to think about it. In the case of a healthy brain, most decisions take place automatically without intervention from the executive system. In the case of someone with dementia, or brain injury, the executive system (or rider) may have even less influence, so when assessing capacity it is necessary to consider how much influence the conscious, executive system still exerts in making a particular decision.

Related to this, it is worth considering something which has been referred to as the frontal lobe paradox (Walsh, 1985). This refers to the dissociation between knowing how to do something and being able to carry it out in practice, which can manifest following impairment of the frontal/executive system (Teuber, 1964). The importance of this was highlighted by George and Gilbert (2018), as someone can score relatively well on tests of executive function but may still demonstrate impaired function in everyday life. It also has implications for assessment of capacity, as someone may appear capacitous based on an interview such as that conducted in the functional test of mental capacity, yet still not be able to be able to apply the requisite decision-making skills in real life. George and Gilbert (2018) highlighted some implications of the frontal lobe paradox for capacity assessments, as most will be undertaken by professionals without specific training in brain injury (and presumably also dementia) which would raise their awareness of the frontal lobe paradox. By relying solely on the interview as set out in the MCA, they may overestimate an individual's ability to live independently or make decisions outside of the interview situation. Cameron and Coding (2020) also drew a distinction between two types of decision: (1) *decisional*, relating to a decision made at a specific point in time, and (2) *decisional and performance*, relating to the ability to apply the information outside of the discussion/interview.

Very little has been written about the implication of the frontal lobe paradox in relation to dementia, although there is some literature in relation to brain injury. Fisher-Hicks, Wood, and Braithwaite (2021) described the case of someone with a frontal lobe injury who would have been considered to have capacity to manage her finances based on the functional test of capacity, yet when her history of financial management was considered, a very different picture emerged. In the case of *TB* v. *KB and LH (Capacity to Conduct Proceedings)* [2019], the capacity of a 75-year-old man with neuropsychological difficulties (the precise cause of which was not specified) was considered in relation to his capacity to litigate. Evidence was presented of deficits in memory, for which compensatory strategies could be employed, and deficits in executive processing, for which it was argued that compensatory strategies were not likely to be effective. Specifically, it was argued that the deficits in executive function would likely mean he would not be able to call to mind the relevant information when required. It was therefore concluded that he did not have capacity to conduct his own litigation.

Therefore, when conducting a capacity assessment on an individual with dementia, it may be necessary to consider whether there is (1) evidence for executive dysfunction, and (2) evidence to suggest that the results of their functional assessment may not be consistent with the person's everyday function.

Deprivation of Liberty and Liberty Protection Safeguards

The MCA draws a distinction between a restriction of liberty, under which all best-interest decisions fall, and a deprivation of liberty, which is more extensive and requires authorisation from an independent body. Deprivation of liberty essentially refers to a form of confinement. The system for this was originally called Deprivation of Liberty Safeguards (DOLS) (Ministry of Justice, 2008), which is to be replace by an amended system called Liberty Protection Safeguards in the Mental Capacity (Amendment) Act 2019. The revised MCA Code of Conduct (draft) p. 252 retains four criteria for determining whether a decision constitutes a restriction or a deprivation of liberty:

1. Freedom to leave. If the person is not able to decide to leave permanently, or to decide where and with whom they wish to live.
2. Continuous supervision and control. They are not left alone for significant periods and cannot make decisions about what they do or where they live.

3. Capacity and consent. A deprivation of liberty only applies if the person has not given 'valid' consent to their confinement. The key term here is 'valid', as a person cannot give consent if they lack the relevant capacity. However, advance consent can be given if it was done so at a point when the person had capacity.

4. It should be noted that DOLS/LPS does not cover medical treatment. An LPS does not give authorisation for the administration of medical treatment to someone who lacks capacity, and indeed a DOLS/LPS authorisation is not required to administer medical treatment to someone who lacks capacity. If medical treatment is required, a capacity assessment specifically related to that treatment is required, most likely followed by a best-interests meeting.

The most influential case law relevant to determining whether a course of action constitutes a restriction of liberty or a deprivation of liberty was two cases which were considered by the UK Supreme Court, and collectively known as Cheshire West (*P* v. *Cheshire West and Chester Council* and *P* v. *Surrey CC* [2014] UKSC 19, [2014] AC 896). Supreme Court Judge Lady Hale identified two relatively simple questions to ask, which she referred to as the 'acid test':

1) Is the person under continuous supervision and control?
2) Are they free to leave?

If the answers are 'yes' to the first question, and 'no' to the second, this constitutes a deprivation of liberty. However, an additional stipulation which was made explicit following these cases was that the important question is not whether the person is asking to leave or objecting to their circumstances, but if they were to ask to leave, would they be permitted to do so? This was extremely important, as prior to this some deprivations of liberty had probably occurred, but independent authorisation had not been sought as the person did not object to their situation and had expressed no desire to leave. The other important outcome of Cheshire West was the acknowledgement that a deprivation of liberty could occur in a community setting, whereas the existing DOLS legislation applied only to hospitals and care homes. This has been addressed in the LPS system, which also covers community settings.

It should be noted that the starting point when applying for LPS is an assessment of mental capacity, as this legislation only applies to people who lack capacity.

The MCA and the Mental Health Act (2007)

The MHA is also a legal framework which may be used in situations which would be considered a deprivation of liberty. The revised MCA Code of Practice acknowledges that there is an interface between LPS and the MHA, but states that 'the interface between these two regimes only occurs in a very small number of specific cases'. However, some people with dementia (and often brain injury) may fall into that interface. The Mental Health Act Code of Practice, paragraph 13.49 states that DOLS and MHA could potentially both be available if:

1. The individual is suffering from a mental disorder (within the meaning of the act)
2. They need to be assessed and/or treated in a hospital for that disorder, or physical conditions related to that disorder
3. The care package may amount to a deprivation of liberty
4. The individual lacks capacity
5. The individual does not object to being admitted to hospital, or to treatment

Table 14.1 Differences between the Mental Capacity Act and the Mental Health Act

Mental Capacity Act	Mental Health Act
Covers all decisions made on behalf of someone who lacks capacity	Applies only to assessment and treatment of someone with a 'mental disorder' in the absence of consent
Applies only if an individual lacks capacity	Mental capacity is not a consideration in most instances. The three exceptions to this are (1) ECT, (2) medication after 3 months of detention, and (3) psychosurgery and hormone treatment
MCA has a clearly defined test of mental capacity	MHA has a less clearly defined definition related to whether they can understand their treatment
If a person has capacity, they can refuse treatment (note that they may have capacity in relation to a specific treatment even if they are not considered to have capacity in relation to their placement and are subject to ILS)	If a person is detained under an MHA section, they cannot refuse treatment for their mental health problem
If someone lacks capacity, they can be treated for a physical health problem (and a mental health problem) if it is considered to be in their best interests	Treatment for physical health problems cannot be enforced under the MHA
The primary consideration under the MCA is whether the person has/lacks capacity	The primary consideration if someone meets the criteria for a mental disorder is whether they constitute a risk to themselves and others
Advanced decisions and LPA must be considered when making a best-interest decision, and can often overrule decisions for treatment	In most cases (other than ECT), the MHA can be applied irrespective of whether there is an advanced decision in place
ILS can be applied in hospitals, care homes, and within the community	Detention under an MHA section can only be done in a hospital or registered mental health unit

Although it is sometimes not that clear which is the appropriate act to apply, Table 14.1 lists some of the key differences between the MCA and the MHA which may be of use when deciding which is the most appropriate legal framework to use.

It should be noted that detention under the MHA is generally considered to be a more serious undertaking with more long-term implications. Consequently, in those cases where either act could apply, MCA/ILS may be selected in preference to an MHA section.

Some Common Capacity Assessments Requested in Dementia, and Some Key Reading Relating to Those Areas (Apart from the Code of Practice)

General Resources

The British Psychological Society has produced a number of documents in relation to mental capacity. Two which are highly useful in all areas, including dementia, are 'What makes a good assessment of capacity?' (British Psychological Society, 2019) and 'Supporting People who Lack Mental Capacity: A Guide to Best Interests Decision Making' (British Psychological Society, 2021).

A useful resource considering different types of capacity assessment can be found in the 'Mental Capacity Casebook: Clinical and Legal Commentary' (Ryan-Morgan, 2019).

Capacity to Make Financial Decisions

This is a question which commonly arises in cases of dementia and encompasses two types of decision. The first is whether someone has capacity to make a specific financial decision (e.g. whether to buy/sell a house). This is a single decision, and assessment of such can be approached in the same way as assessing for any other single decision. The second type of decision is usually phrased in terms of whether or not someone is capable of managing their finances. This requires a somewhat more extensive assessment as financial decisions range from relatively simple, such as whether to purchase a cup of coffee, to highly complex, such as how to invest large sums of money. Newby and Ryan-Morgan (2013) recommend that this is not seen in binary terms, but advocate considering decision-making as a continuum of complexity relating to property and affairs. Empowerment Matters (2014) published a comprehensive guide to assessing capacity for financial decisions, giving examples of questions for how to approach each level of decision-making.

Deciding on Care and Residence

This is a very common question asked in relation to individuals with dementia. If asked whether they would wish to remain living in their own home or consider alternatives, many people will choose the former. However, when someone develops dementia, the question arises of whether they can safely remain in their current circumstances, either independently or with the support of carers, or whether a higher level of support is required, such as that found in residential or nursing home settings. The question often arises in the context of a hospital admission, following which assessments are required to ensure a safe discharge.

When undertaking an assessment of this nature, some caution must be retained with regards to determining whether someone can weigh up the advantages and disadvantages of remaining at home, as it is common for people not to see or acknowledge any disadvantages. It may therefore be necessary to proceed by ascertaining whether they have a realistic appreciation of their care needs, and whether these can be met in their current living situation. It may also be necessary to consider the distinction between knowing and doing (Teuber, 1964), and to consider the evidence for how well they were previously coping and whether there has been any significant change which may impact upon their coping ability.

Capacity to Decide on Medical Treatment

The MCA covers capacity to consent to medical treatment. When assessing capacity, it is important to ascertain whether the person has a full understanding of not only the treatment being proposed, but also possible treatment alternatives. The person may also have made an advanced decision to refuse certain treatments. This must be in writing if the treatment is life-sustaining. Ryan-Morgan (2019) highlights several areas which cannot be covered by an advanced decision: refusal of pain relief, food, drink, warmth, or nursing care. The advanced decision cannot specify a particular treatment, cannot request assisted death, and cannot refuse treatment under the Mental Health Act (2007).

Capacity to Decide on Making A Will

Many people who experience cognitive decline will have made a will before this occurs. However, there will be some cases of people who wish to make a will because there was not a previous one in place, and there will also be cases where someone wishes to draft a new will which differs significantly from a previous one. The question which arises will therefore be whether someone has capacity (referred to as testamentary capacity) at the time they make or change a will?

In addition to the MCA Code of Practice, there are other guidelines often cited in relation to this issue. A legal test for testamentary capacity was set out in *Banks* v. *Goodfellow* (1870) LR 5 QB 549, 565, which specified the testator should:

1. Understand the nature and effects of making a will
2. Understand the extent of the property of which they are disposing
3. Comprehend and appreciate the claims to which he ought to give effect
4. Not be affected by any disorder of mind or 'insane delusion'

The MCA adds to this that the testator needs to understand and evaluate the reasonably foreseeable consequences of the will. The burden of proof also differs in the MCA, as it begins with the presumption of capacity meaning which must be rebutted, whereas *Banks* v. *Goodfellow* requires proof that the testator had the necessary capacity to make the will.

The 'Golden Rule' is also frequently cited, which was set out by Mr Justice Templeman in the case of *Kenward* v. *Adams*: ChD 29 Nov 1975, which is the requirement for an aged or previously unwell testator to have capacity and understanding established by a medical practitioner. However, as Ryan-Morgan (2019) points out, the Golden Rule is a statement of good practice rather than a legal rule.

Whether the MCA has replaced the *Banks* v. *Goodfellow* (1870) legal test of capacity was considered in the appeal of the case of *Clitheroe* v. *Bond* (2020) EWHC 1185 (ch), where Mrs. Justice Falk ruled that *Banks* v. *Goodfellow* (1870) has not been over-ridden by the MCA.

Capacity to Grant Power of Attorney

As explained earlier, OPA is granted by someone who has capacity, and is invalid should they lose capacity. Lasting POA is granted by someone who has capacity is anticipation of a situation arising whereby they may lose capacity, and only comes into force should that situation occur. The question which may often arise in cases of dementia is whether someone who has not established an ordinary or lasting POA has the capacity to do so. A capacity assessment would be required in such cases.

Appendix L   Case Studies

Case Study: Mrs B

Mrs B was a 75-year-old female with a diagnosis of vascular dementia following a series of relatively minor strokes, the most recent of which had left her with an unsafe swallow. She was in hospital under a DOLS authorisation. Mrs B had made a good physical recovery from each stroke, although she had some mild limitations on her mobility. Speech and language therapy (SLT) had assessed her swallow as unsafe and recommended she should not take food or drink orally, instead using a tube inserted through the abdominal wall into the stomach. Mrs. B also underwent various medical investigations, all of which also indicated she had an unsafe swallow and was at risk of aspirational pneumonia, which was demonstrated when she chose not to follow advice and ate some snacks furtively brought in by her partner.

Mrs B underwent some cognitive testing, which revealed well-preserved memory ability, good communication, but deficits in speed of information processing and executive processing, all of which were consistent with the diagnosis of vascular dementia. As Mrs B was adamant she wished to continue to take food and drink orally against advice, it was decided to undertake a capacity assessment in relation to this. This also had implications for her DOLS authorisation, as she made it clear that should she be discharged, she would eat and drink normally.

Mrs B was considered to meet the criteria for the diagnostic test and went on to undertake the functional test. It was clear she understood the relevant information, could retain it, and was able to communicate her decision. However, when asked to weigh up information, she demonstrated a very rigid thinking style. Specifically, she rejected the conclusions of the medical and SLT assessments, stating that the difficulties with her swallow were caused by a lack of practice as she had been nil by mouth since her most recent stroke. She was adamant that it would improve if she were allowed to start consuming food and drink orally, despite experiencing several episodes of aspirational pneumonia when she had tried. The outcome of the initial capacity assessment was that, on the balance of probabilities, Mrs B. did not have the capacity to make this decision. Mrs B objected to this conclusion, as did her partner, which led to the request for a second opinion.

During the second opinion assessment, Mrs B's partner was interviewed, along with some of her friends, all of whom were consistent in stating that Mrs B's very rigid reasoning style was typical of her long-term personality, and not something which had developed following her brain injury. The second opinion assessor concluded that the criteria for the diagnostic test had been met, and that her reasoning suggested she could not evaluate the relevant information as assessed by the functional test. However, it had not been established that Mrs B's rigid reasoning and rejection of medical and SLT opinion was a result of the stroke. The conclusion was that the causative nexus had not been sufficiently established, and consequently there was not sufficient evidence to rebut the presumption of capacity.

Case Study: Mr W

Mr W was a 72-year-old male with a diagnosis of probable dementia of the Alzheimer type and a long-term history of depression predating the onset of cognitive decline by several decades. Mr W lived with his wife, who reported that his depression had worsened considerably and she was finding it difficult to meet his needs as a result. As Mr W had been taking an anti-depressant intermittently for several years, it was questioned whether a change of medication might confer some benefits. Mr W was adamant that he would not accept a change in medication, therefore it was questioned whether he had capacity to make this decision. A previous capacity assessment approximately a year earlier had concluded that he had capacity to decide on medication; however, it was argued by his wife that his reasoning had declined significantly due to a combination of worsening cognition and possibly also in relation to worsening mood.

Mr W was apparently agreeable to take his dementia-related medication (an ACE inhibitor) and did not refuse his already-prescribed anti-depressant medication, but was unwilling to try a change of medication. A second capacity assessment was arranged on the basis that there had been a probable decline in cognitive ability and an increase in the severity of his depression. Part of the assessment included an administration of the ACE-III, which indicated a decline in overall score from 75/100 to 65/100. Mr W was no longer engaging in activities, and would frequently neglect personal care, not showering or changing his clothes for several days. This represented a significant change in his day-to-day function, but it was not clear whether this could be attributed to progression of dementia or lowering of mood.

Mr W consented to the assessment and was seen at home. He had a good understanding of what his current medication consisted of, and the intended purpose of his anti-depressant medication. When asked whether he considered his current anti-depressant to be effective, he stated he did not consider this to be the case. When asked if he would consider trying an alternative, he stated very clearly that he would not, his reason being that anti-depressants do not work. This appeared contradictory as he was willing to continue with his current medication, which he stated did not work, but would not try an alternative. Mr W declined to engage with this discussion, instead repeatedly stating 'they don't work, none of them work'. This very rigid thinking style was not considered to be a personality trait and had not been apparent during his previous capacity assessment, which had been in relation to commencing his original anti-depressant medication. His wife volunteered that this was characteristic of his depression, and this was typical of how he responded when his mood was low.

It was concluded that Mr W did not have capacity to decide on his medication, and a best-interest meeting was arranged which included the prescribing psychiatrist, his GP, Mr W's wife, an IMCA, and a representative from the Alzheimer's Society who knew Mr W and his wife as they accessed support from this service. Although there was agreement that Mr W did not have capacity, there was not absolute agreement that a change of medication would necessarily bring about a change in his mood. Mr W's wife was very much in favour of a change of prescription; however, it was pointed out that there was little published evidence for greater effectiveness of one anti-depressant over another, although there was evidence from single case studies and the psychiatrist had observed improvement within the context of their own practice. It was also pointed out that the changes which had occurred over the last year may be in part related to progression of his dementia. Careful consideration was given to whether the new medication had any possible risks or ill-effects, and this was considered not to be the case. It was ultimately decided to trial a different medication, and there were no obvious ill-effects and some possible benefits.

References

British Psychological Society (2019). What makes a good assessment of capacity? www.bps.org.uk/guideline/what-makes-good-assessment-capacity.

British Psychological Society (2021). Supporting people who lack mental capacity: A guide to best interests decision making. www.bps.org.uk/guideline/supporting-people-who-lack-mental-capacity-guide-best-interests-decision-making.

Cameron, J., & Codling, J. (2020). When mental capacity assessments must delve beneath what people say to what they do. *Community Care.* www.communitycare.co.uk/2020/10/28/mental-capacity-assessments-must-delve-beneath-people-say/.

Department for Constitutional Affairs (2007). Mental Capacity Act (2005): Code of Practice. www.gov.uk/government/publications/mental-capacity-act-code-of-practice.

Department for Constitutional Affairs (2007). *Mental Capacity Act 2005: Code of Practice.* London: The Stationary Office.

Empowerment Matters (2014). Making financial decisions: Guidance for assessing, supporting and empowering specific decision making. https://empowermentmattersweb.files.wordpress.com/2014/09/assessing-capacity-financial-decisions-guidance-final.pdf.

Farmer, T. (2017). *Grandpa on a Skateboard* (2nd edn). Great Britain: Rethink Press.

Fisher-Hicks, S., Wood, R., & Braithwaite, B. (2021). The Frontal lobe paradox. In P. Moore, S. Brifcani & A. Worthington (Eds), *Neuropsychological Aspects of Brain Injury Litigation* (pp. 140–57). London: Routledge.

George, M., & Gilbert, S. (2018). Mental Capacity Act (2005) Assessments: Why everyone needs to know about the frontal lobe paradox. *The Neuropsychologist,* **5,** 59–66.

Haidt, J. (2006). *The Happiness Hypothesis: Finding Modern Truth in Ancient Wisdom.* New York: Basic Books.

Haidt, J. (2012). *The Righteous Mind: Why Good People are Divided by Politics and Religion.* New York: Pantheon.

Ministry of Justice (2008). *Mental Capacity Act 2005 Deprivation of Liberty Safeguards: Code of Practice to Supplement the Main Mental Capacity Act 2005 Code of Practice.* London: TSO.

Newby, H., & Ryan-Morgan, T. (2013). Assessment of mental capacity. In G. Newby, R. Coetzer, A. Disley & S. Wetherhead (Eds.), *The Handbook of Real Neuropsychological Rehabilitation in Acquired Brain Injury* (pp. 179–207). London: Karnac.

Ryan-Morgan, T. (2019). *Mental Capacity Casebook: Clinical and Legal Commentary.* London: Routledge.

Teuber, H. L. (1964). The riddle of the frontal lobe function in man. In J. M. Warren & K. Akert (Eds.), *The Frontal Granular Cortex and Behaviour* (pp. 410–58). New York: McGraw-Hill.

Walsh, K. W. (1985). *Understanding Brain Damage: A Primer of Neuropsychological Evaluation.* London: Churchill Livingstone.

Index

Aarsland, D., 90, 91
ACB Calculator website, 23
acetylcholinesterase inhibitors
(AChE inhibitors),
see also under
pharmacological
interventions, 140–3
acquired brain injury,
processes, 121–2
Addenbrookes Cognitive
Evaluation (ACE-III),
18, 66, 108
case studies, 26, 99
cut-off score, 21
identification of PCA, 66
Advanced Cognitive Training
for Independent and
Vital Elderly (ACTIVE
study), 134
age
as risk factor for developing
dementia, 5–6
average age of onset for
different dementia
types, *5*
agnosia, 38, 111
Aguirre, E., 135
Ahlskog, J. E., 151
Albert, 20, 89
alcohol consumption
abstention from and
recovery of function, 35,
122, 123
relationship with
dementia, 150
alcohol-induced
neurocognitive
disorder, *see also*
alcohol-related brain
damage (ARBD), 121
alcohol-related brain damage
(ARBD)
overview, 121
acquired brain injury,
processes, 121–2
age of onset, 121
case study, 127

classification
as brain injury, 122
as dementia, 122
cognitive sequelae, 124
diagnostic criteria, 125
ethanol-related
neurotoxicity and, 123
neuropsychological
assessment, timing, 126
prevalence, 121
thiamine deficiency and, 123
toxic processes at work, 123
key points, 126–7
see also alcohol-related
dementia; Korsakoff's
dementia;
Wernicke–Korsakoff's
syndrome (WKS)
alcohol-related dementia, 3
Aldridge, G. M., 91
Alexander, G. E., 106
Almeida, O. P., 151
Almeida-Meza, P., 9
Alzheimer, Alois, 5, 61
Alzheimer's disease
overview, 59
AChE inhibitors licensed for
use in the UK, 141
amyloid cascade
hypothesis, 62
atypical presentations, 66
frontal variant DAT
(fvDAT), 67
limbic-predominant age-
related TDP-43
encephalopathy
(LATE), 67
logopenic variant primary
progressive aphasia
(lvPPA), 67
more commonly found in
YOAD, 61
posterior cortical atrophy
(PCA), 38, 66, 68, *161*
autosomal dominant familial
DAT, 61
case studies, 68–9

comorbidities, 59, 94
comparison of young-onset
and late-onset, 61
continuum of
progression, 61
diagnostic criteria, 63–4
ATN system, 63
exclusion criteria, 64
diagnostic tests for, 65–6
DSM-V criteria, 64
fluid biomarkers, 162
genetic risk factors, 6
genetics, 63
neuropsychological
assessment, 64–5
pathology, 61, 63
PCA and, 38
percentage of cases with
comorbid Parkinson's
disease, 4
percentage of cases with
vascular pathology,
4, 149
prevalence and incidence,
59–61
relationship with
dementia, 61
stages, *62*
typical life expectancy, 61
VCI and (mixed
dementia), 75–6
key points, 68
Amieva, H., 134
amyloid cascade hypothesis,
62
Anang, J. B., 90
anomia, 111
anterograde amnesia, 39, 65,
68, 124
apathy, as potential effect of
damage to the anterior
cingulate cortex, 42
Arts, N., 123,
125
α-synuclein protein, 4
atrial fibrillation, as risk factor
for dementia, 149, 150

atrophy, patterns of associated
with cause of
dementia, *161*
attention
APA definition, 40
cognitive processes and
associated circuits, 40–1

Bäckman, L., 65
Banks v. *Goodfellow*,
testamentary
capacity, 175
Barresi, B., 112
Bartels, C., 151
base rates, the concept of in
psychology, 51–2
Beach, T. G., 15
Benson, D. F., 65
Beynon, R., 23
biomarkers
Alzheimer's disease, 63, 162
ATN system, 63
definition and role in
classification of
dementia, 159
fluid biomarkers, 162
imaging
functional, SPECT and
PET, 161–2
structural, CT and MRI,
159–60
in clinical practice, 162
key points, 163
blood pressure, relationship
with development of
dementia, 149
blood supply
and reduction of dementia
risk, 149–50, 152
dementia risk reduction
strategies, 149–50
impact of compromised
blood supply to the
brain, 7
see also vascular cognitive
impairment/dementia
(VCI/VaD)
blood, biomarkers for possible
causes of cognitive
decline, *24*
Bonhoeffer, Karl, *122*
Bora, E., 109
Boston Diagnostic Aphasia
Examination, 112
Boston Naming Test, 112

Bournewood case, mental
capacity, 165
Boustani, M., 23
Braak, H., 87
Bradshaw, J., 93
bradykinesia, 87
brain cells
effects of toxic agents on, 3
impact of loss of blood
supply to the brain on, 7
pruning process, 8
brain organisation
role of circuits, 34
see also cerebral
organisation; functional
neuroanatomy
brain, sagittal view, *41*
Braithwaite, B., 171
Brayne, C., 90, 92
Breakspeare, M., 34
Bredesen, D., 153
Broca's aphasia, 38, 112
Brockhaus, R., 55
Broe, M., 107
Brooks, B. L., 51
Brown, Derren, 133
Buckley, J., 141

Cadar, D., 9
CADASIL, 7, 77, 80
Caine, D., 125
California Verbal Learning
test, 65
Cameron, J., 76, 171
cannabis, relationship with
dementia, 150
capacity, *see* mental capacity.
cerebral amyloid angiopathy,
61, 76
cerebral organisation
general principles, 36
see also functional
neuroanatomy
Chan, P. C., 93
Charles Bonnet syndrome,
DLB and, 94
Children's Act (2004), 168
cholesterol levels, and
development of
dementia, 149
chronic heart failure,
association with
cognitive decline, 23
chronic pain, association with
cognitive decline, 23

'circuit disorders', use of the
term, 36
circumin, 153
Clare, L., 135
Clinical Dementia Rating
(CDR), 21
Clitheroe v. *Bond*, testamentary
capacity, 175
Codling, J., 171
cognition, Neisser's
definition, 37
Cognitive Ageing and Function
Studies (Matthews
et al.), 1
cognitive decline, possible
explanations other than
dementia, 22–3
cognitive impairment,
establishing evidence
for, 18–20
screening instruments, 18–20
cognitive processes and
associated circuits, 37–42
attention, 40–1
brain, sagittal view, *41*
emotion/affect, 42
executive function, 41–2
language, 38–9
memory, 39–40
memory, Papez circuit, *40*
perception, 38
cognitive rehabilitation
overview, 131
aim of, 132
cognitive stimulation, 135
cognitive training
exercises, 134
healthy older adult, MCI
and dementia, 134–5
compensation, 131, 134
effectiveness with dementia,
evidence for, 134
environmental modification,
131, 134
effectiveness, 135
external memory aids
and, 133
evidence of effectiveness,
considerations, 135–6
ICF framework, 131–2
memory rehabilitation
external memory aids, 133
internal memory strategies,
132–3
key points, 136

cognitive reserve, 8, 9, 151
cognitive stimulation, 131, 151
cognitive training, 131, 134–5, 136, 153
compensation, 131
confabulation
    DLB and, 94
    Korsakoff's syndrome and, *122*, 123, 124
confrontation naming deficits, 66
connectomics, 9, 34
corticobasal degeneration (CBD), 96, 97
classification, 86
court-appointed deputies, 169
Courtney, C., 142
Crawford, S., 54
Crutch, S. J., 66
Cummings, J. L., 65, 90, 143

Dean, A., 54
dedifferentiation, meaning of, 34
delirium, as possible explanation for cognitive decline, 22
dementia
    assessment challenges, 54–5
    definition, 1, 122
    global benefits of delaying onset, 148
    pharmacological interventions, rate of development, 148
    prevalence and incidence in the UK, 1
dementia of the Alzheimer's type (DAT)
    comorbidity with DLB, 59
    comparison with WKS, *126*
    menopause and, 59–60
    see also Alzheimer's disease
Dementia Severity Rating Scale (DSRS), 21
dementia with Lewy bodies (DLB)
    age of onset and progression, 92
    comorbidity with Alzheimer's pathology, 94
    comorbidity with DAT, 59
    comparison with PDD, 89–90, 92, 94, *95*
    diagnostic criteria, 93–4

distinguishing Alzheimer's disease from, 24
DLB-MCI, 94
genetics, 95
hallucinations, confabulations and Charles Bonnet syndrome, 94
imaging, role of, 97–8, 161
key diagnostic features, 64
prevalence and incidence, 92
relationship with PCA, 66
response to medication, 96
sleep disorders in, 93
SPECT and diagnosis of, 161
toxic agent, 89
demyelination, 35
depression
    as 'circuit disorder', 36
    relationship with dementia, 151
Deprivation of Liberty Safeguards (DOLS), *see also* Liberty Protection Safeguards (LPS), 165
deprivation of liberty, *Cheshire West* case, 172
diabetes, as risk factor for dementia, 150
diagnosis
    formulation and, 15
    the definition, 15
diagnosis of dementia
    biomarkers, 9, 159
    case studies, 25–8
    cognitive testing, appropriate use, 18, 19
    context establishment, 15
    relevant information, *16*
    see also risk factors for developing dementia
    dementia checklist, 29
    diagnostic process, 17–20
    differential diagnosis, 2, 9
    DSM-V criteria, 2, 20, 50
    evidence for cognitive impairment, 18–20
    screening instruments, 18–20
    expert and novice differences, 15, *16*
    functional decline
        distinguishing between MCI and dementia, 20
        establishing, 20, *21*

identifying the subtype, 2–3
imaging, 9, 23–5
MCI/dementia decision tree, 25
neuropsychological assessment, 18–19
other possible explanations for cognitive decline, 22–3
    blood markers for other possible causes, *24*
    delirium, 22
    medical problems, 23
    medications, 22–3
    mental health problems, 22
    psychosis, 22
    sensory impairment, 23
post-mortem confirmation, 15
screening instruments, 18–20, 21
severity, 21
    DSM-V classification, 21
    screening instruments, 21
key points, 25
diaschisis, meaning of, 34
diet, and reduction of dementia risk, 152
dietary supplements, and improved cognition, 153
differential diagnosis, importance of, 2, 9
dopamine, role of in Parkinson's disease, 86, 96
dorsal stream, 38
    example of selective impairment to, 38
dorsolateral prefrontal cortex
    function, 41
    location, *41*
Draper, B., 121
Dubois, B., 87
d'Ydewalle, G., 124
dyspraxia, 66

efficacy, vs effectiveness, 139
Effort Scale (ES), 54
Ekman faces, 109
emotion/affect, cognitive processes and associated circuits, 42
Empowerment Matters, 174

encephalopathy, Wernicke's
  description, *122*
episodic memory, 39–40
errorless learning, 132, 133
Evans, J. J., 54
executive function, cognitive
  processes and associated
  circuits, 41–2
exercise, and reduction of
  dementia risk, 151

Farmer, T., 168
Feldman, H. H., 51
Finnish Geriatric Intervention
  Study to Prevent
  Cognitive Impairment
  (FINGER), 153
Fisher-Hicks, S., 171
Fornito, A., 9
Fox, N., 143
frontal lobe paradox, 170–1
frontotemporal
  dementia (FTD)
  overview, 105
  behavioural variant
    (bvFTD), 106–7
    cognitive assessment, 109
    diagnostic criteria, 108
    exclusion criteria, 108
    pattern of atrophy, 107
  case studies, 116
  cognitive assessment, 108–9
  diagnostic features, 64
  genetics and other risk
    factors, 106
  percentage having a vascular
    component, 149
  prevalence and
    incidence, 105
  toxic agent, 106
  key points, 115
  see also primary progressive
    aphasia (PPA)
functional decline
  distinguishing between MCI
    and dementia, 20
  establishing, 20, *21*
functional imaging, SPECT
  and PET, 161–2
functional neuroanatomy
  amygdala, 35, 42
  anterior cingulate cortex,
    41, 42
  axons, 34
  basal ganglia, 35
  cerebellum, 36

circuits, 34
cognitive processes and
  associated circuits, 37–42
  attention, 40–1
  brain, sagittal view, *41*
  emotion/affect, 42
  executive function, 41–2
  language, 38–9
  memory, 39–40
  memory, Papez circuit, *40*
  perception, 38
cortex, 36–7
  basal ganglia in relation
    to, *36*
  motor and sensory organs
    of, *37*
  dendrites, 34
  frontal lobe, position of, 36
  glial cells, role of, 8, 34
  grey matter and white
    matter, 35–6
  illustration of synapse and
    neuron, *140*
  motor cortex, location, 36
  neurons, 34
  orbitofrontal cortex,
    function and location,
    41, 41
  parietal lobe, and integration
    of sensory
    information, 36
  primary sensory cortex, 36
  primary visual cortex, 36
  thalamus, effects of damage
    to, 35
  ventromedial prefrontal
    cortex, 42
  key points, 42

Galvin, R., 121
Gao, S., 60
Gates, N., 134
George, M., 171
Gerhand, S., 55
Gilbert, S., 171
Gilchrist, G., 121
Ginkgo Biloba, 153
Gitlin, L. N., 135
glymphatic system, as risk
  factor for developing
  dementia, 8
Goodglass, H., 112
Gorno-Tempini, M. L., 67, 110
Goulding, P. J., 111
Green, P., 55
Grossman, M., 67

Hachinski Ischemic Scale,
  76, 80
Hacker, D., 55
Haidt, J., 170
hallucinations, DLB and, 94
Harding, L., 124
Harper, C. G., 121, 124
Harper, L., 24, 160
Harvey, R. J., 121
hearing loss, association with
  increased risk of
  developing dementia,
  23
Hely, M. A., 90
Herbert, V., 77
Hill, N. T., 134
Hillis, A. E., 67
hippocampal sclerosis, 59, *161*
Holdnack, J. A., 51
Hospital Anxiety and
  Depression Scale
  (HADS), 22
Howard, R., 142
Hughes, T. A., 90
Huntington's disease (HD),
  7, 88

imaging
  and diagnosis of dementia,
    9, 23–5
  functional, SPECT and PET,
    161–2
  role of in diagnosing DLB,
    PDD and atypical
    Parkinsonian
    disorders, 97–8
  structural, CT and MRI,
    159–60
incidence, definition, 1
inflammation
  as risk factor for developing
    dementia, 8
  proteinopathies and, 76
International Classification
  of Functioning,
  Disability and Health
  (ICF), cognitive
  rehabilitation
  framework, 131–2
ischaemic stroke, 7
Iverson, G. L., 51, 55
Iwagami, M., 149

Jack, C. R., 63
Janvin, C. C., 88, 91
Jones, C. A., 55

Kaduszkiewicz, H., 142
Kaplan, E., 65, 112
Katzman, R., 8
Kaufman Assessment Battery
    for Children, 49
Keane, J., 108
Kelley, B. J., 5
Kenward v. *Adams*,
    testamentary
    capacity, 175
Kertesz, A., 109
Kiloh, L. G., 121
King, Rebecca, 23
Kipps, C. M., 109
Korsakoff, Sergei, *122*
Korsakoff's dementia, 121, 122
Korsakoff's syndrome, *see also*
    Wernicke's
    encephalopathy;
    Wernicke–Korsakoff's
    syndrome (WKS), *122*,
    123, 124
Kril, J. J., 121, 124
Kuru, mechanism of
    infectivity, 6

Lagarde, J., 97
language
    cognitive processes and
        associated circuits, 38–9
    lateralisation and, 38
lasting power of attorney,
    169, 175
late-onset Alzheimer's disease
    (LOAD), 61
lateralisation
    cerebral organisation and, 36
    language and, 38
Leach, L., 65
letter fluency, 65
Lewy bodies
    and MSA, 86
    as hallmark of Parkinson's
        disease, 4
    in LOAD and YOAD, 61
    infective process
        hypothesis, 87
    inter-related disorders
        associated with, 86
    progression of, 87
    role of in Parkinson's disease
        and other Parkinsonian
        disorders, 86–7
Lewy body dementia, *see*
    dementia with Lewy
    bodies (DLB).

Lewy body disorders, and
    AChE inhibitors, 142
Leyton, C. E., 114
Liberty Protection
    Safeguards (LPS)
    interface with MHA, 172
    introduction of the
        concept, 165
Liberty Protection Safeguards
    in the Mental Capacity
    (Amendment) Act
    (2019), 171
Liebman, J., 135
Lim, C., 4
list learning tests, 65
Litvan, I., 88, *89*
Loy, C. T., 7
Luria, A., 133

Major Neurocognitive
    Disorder, 2, 76, 79, 121
Marshall, C. R., 112
Mathuranath, P. S., 108
Matsunaga, S., 142
Matthews, F. E., 1
McCracken, C., 92
McGuire, C., 54
McShane, 143
Medical Symptom Validity
    Test (MSVT), 54
Meehl, P. E., 51
Meier, M. H., 150
memory
    cerebral organisation and, 36
    cognitive processes and
        associated circuits,
        39–40
memory rehabilitation
    external memory aids, 133
    internal memory strategies,
        132–3
menopause, relationship with
    DAT pathology, 59–60
mental capacity
    advanced decision to refuse
        certain treatments, 175
    and lasting power of
        attorney, 169, 175
    assessments, appropriate
        persons, 166
    care and residence
        decisions, 174
    case studies, 176–7
    causative nexus, 168
    CMSL threshold, 168, 169
    cognitive testing, 169

consent to medical
    treatment, 175
dementia and the frontal
    lobe paradox, 170–1
diagnostic test, 168
elephant and rider
    analogy, 170
financial decisions, 174
fluctuating capacity, 170
functional test, 168
key considerations, 165–6
meaning of, 165
power of attorney and court-
    appointed deputies, 169
TB v. *KB and LH*, 171
testamentary capacity, 175
the Mental Capacity Act
    (2005), 165
    see also Mental Capacity
        Act (MCA)
useful resources, 174
Mental Capacity Act (MCA,
    2005)
    and the Mental Health Act
        (MHA), 172–3
    Bournewood case, 165
    capacity in childhood,
        168
    decisions covered by, 167
    decisions not covered by,
        167
    differences between MHA
        and, *173*
    historical development, 165
    Independent Mental
        Capacity Advocate
        (IMCA), 169
    Liberty Protection
        Safeguards amendment
        published, 165
    liberty, restriction vs
        deprivation, 171–2
    principles of, 166–7
    scope of application, 165
    test components, 168
Mental Health Act (MHA,
    1983), 167, 172–3
Mestre, H., 8
Mesulam, M.-M., 110–11
Mild Cognitive Impairment
    (MCI), 20
    assessment challenges, 54–5
    distinction between
        dementia and in terms
        of function, 20
    DSM-V criteria, 50

(MCI) (cont.)
  Parkinson's disease Mild
    Cognitive Impairment
    (PD-MCI), 88–9
  pharmacological
    interventions, rate of
    development, 148
  prevalence, 1
Mild Neurocognitive Disorder,
  2, 64
Minor Neurocognitive
  Disorder, 20
mixed dementia
  and AChE inhibitors, 142
  diagnostic challenges, 4
  meaning of, 59, 74
  pathology, 75–6
mnemonics, 53, 131,
  132–3, 134
modularity, theory of, 46
Moerman-van den Brink,
  W. G., 124
Montijo, J., 55
Montreal Cognitive
  Assessment (MoCA),
  18, 27, 88, 91
Mori, Y., 8
Morley, S., 52
Morris, M. C., 152
Morrison, G. S., 121
Mosimann, U. P., 94
Multi-Domain Alzheimer
  Preventative trial
  (MAPT), France, 153
multi-infarct dementia, 75,
  76, 79
multiple sclerosis, 35, 79,
  162
multiple systems atrophy
  (MSA), 96
  Lewy bodies and, 86
  toxic agent, 89, 96
myelin, impact of damage
  to, 34

National Adult Reading Test
  (NART), as tool for
  estimating premorbid
  ability, 89
Neary, D., 107, 111
Nedergaard, M., 8
Neisser, U., 37
Nelson, P. T., 68
neuroanatomy, functional, see
  functional
  neuroanatomy.

neuron, illustration of synapse
  and, 140
neuropsychological assessment
  Alzheimer's disease, 64–5
  appropriate use, 18–19
  aspects of cognitive function
    to cover, 53
  assessing when required, 45
  base rates, 51–2
  bvFTD, 109
  evaluating change, 52
  formulas and calculations, 56
  FTD, 108
  performance validity, 54–5
  premorbid ability,
    estimating, 50–1
  psychometrics, and normal
    distribution, 47, 47, 48
  scores
    recognising
      significance, 50
    types of, 48–50
  suitable assessors, 45
  test selection, 53
  timing, 126
  underlying assumptions, 46
  key points, 55
Newby, H., 174
Niu, H., 59
Non-verbal Medical Symptom
  Validity Test, 54

obesity
  as risk factor for
    dementia, 150
  association with FTD, 106
object recognition, role of the
  ventral stream, 38
O'Brien, J. T., 143
occipital lobes, 36–8
Omega-3 fish oils, 153
ordinary power of attorney
  (OPA), 169
Orrell, M., 135
Owen, A. M., 135

paired associate learning
  (PAL), 65
Papez circuit, 39, 40
Papua New Guinea, 6
Parkinsonian disorders
  overview, 139
  atypical, 96
    imaging and, 97–8
  case studies, 99
  diagnostic criteria, 97–8

role of the Lewy body, 86
  key points, 98
  see also individual disorders
Parkinson's disease (PD)
  age of onset, 87
  and the substantia
    nigra, 86–7
  as 'circuit disorder', 36
  cognitive changes with, 87–8
  diagnostic criteria, 87–8
  Lewy bodies as hallmark of, 4
  pathology, 86–7
  prevalence, 86
  response to medication, 96
  SPECT and diagnosis of, 161
Parkinson's disease
    dementia (PDD)
  classification, 88
  cognitive profile associated
    with, 91
  comorbidity with
    Alzheimer's
    pathology, 94
  comparison with DLB,
    89–90, 94, 95
  diagnostic criteria, 91–2
  genetics, 95
  imaging, role of, 97–8
  predictive factors, 90–1
  prevalence and incidence, 90
  response to medication, 96
  toxic agent, 89
Parkinson's disease Mild
    Cognitive Impairment
    (PD-MCI), 88–9
  diagnostic criteria, 89
  perception, cognitive processes
    and associated
    circuits, 38
Performance Validity Tests
  (PVTs), 54
Petersen, R. C., 41
pharmacological interventions
  overview, 109
  AChE inhibitors
    overview, 140
    and non-Alzheimer's
      dementia, 142
    and nursing home
      care, 142
    effectiveness, 141
    licensed for use in the
      UK, 141
    placebo effects, 142
    side effects, 142
  aducanumab, 139, 143

clinical trials, types of, 145
disease-modifying
    treatments
    overview, 143
    comparison with
        symptom-modifying
        treatments, 139
    mode of action, 143–4
    plaques, tangles and
        amyloid oligomers, 144
    donanemab, 144
    donepezil, 141, 142
    efficacy vs effectiveness, 139
    galantamine, 141, 143
    memantine, 139, 142–3
    rate of development, 148
    rivastigmine, 141
    key points, 145
Phongpreecha, T., 91
physical exercise, and
    reduction of dementia
    risk, 151
Pick's disease, see also
    frontotemporal
    dementia (FTD), 106
Pillon, B., 87
Pirozzolo, F. J., 87
positron emission tomography
    (PET), 161–2
Posner, M. I., 41
posterior cortical atrophy
    (PCA), 38, 66, 68, 161
power of attorney (POA), 169
prefrontal cortex, function, 36
prevalence, definition, 1
Prevention of Dementia by
    Intensive Vascular Care
    (PreDIVA),
    Netherlands, 153
Price, C. C., 75
primary progressive
    aphasia (PPA)
    overview, 86
    clinical features of
        subtypes, 114
    diagnostic criteria, 110–11
    disease progression, 110
    genetics, 109
    logopenic variant
        (lvPPA), 113
    non-fluent variant (nfvPPA),
        112–13
    prevalence, 109
    relationship with classical
        stroke-based
        models, 109
    semantic variant
        (svPPA), 112

key points, 115
Prince, M., 1
procedural learning,
    Korsakoff's syndrome
    and, 124
progressive supranuclear palsy
    (PSP), 97
    classification, 86
prosopagnosia, 38, 66
proteinopathies
    associated forms of
        dementia, 4
    inflammation and, 76
    meaning of, 3
    PPA and, 109
psychology, key role in
    reducing risk of
    dementia, 149
psychometrics
    and normal distribution, 47,
        47, 48
    meaning of, 46
psychosis, as possible
    explanation for
    cognitive decline, 22

Rabino, Steve, 23
Ramos, E. M., 109
Ratnavalli, E., 105
Reality Orientation, 135
ReCODE protocol, 153
rehearsal strategies, 132
reliable change index, 52, 56, 89
Reliable Digit Span, 54
reminiscence therapy, 134
Rensen, Y. C., 124
Repeatable Battery for the
    Assessment of
    Neuropsychological
    Status (RBANS),
    52, 53–4
respiratory disease, association
    with cognitive
    decline, 23
retrograde amnesia, 39, 65, 124
Rey Auditory Learning Test, 65
Rey's Dot Counting Test, 54
rheumatoid arthritis,
    association with
    cognitive decline, 23
Richardson's syndrome, 97
risk factors for developing
    dementia
    age, 5–6
    blood supply, 7
    risk reduction strategies,
        149–50
    genetics and epigenetics, 6–7

glymphatic system, 8
hearing loss, 23
inflammation, 8
Livingston's list, 148
reducing
    overview, 148–9
    alcohol, 150
    cannabis, 150
    depression, 151
    programmes aimed at, 153
    psychology, key role, 149
    ReCODE protocol, 153
    sleep disturbance, 152
    through cognitive
        stimulation, 151
    through diet, 152
    through physical
        exercise, 151
    through social
        engagement, 152
    tobacco use, 150
    vascular risk factors,
        149–50, 152
    with dietary supplements
        and medications, 153
    key points, 154
sleep disturbance, 8
reducing risk, 152
Ritchie, K., 121
Rogalski, E., 110
Rosen, A., 51
Rosso, S. M., 106
Ryan-Morgan, T., 174–5

Sachdev, P. S., 75, 77
Sagan, Carl, 135
Saling, M., 93
Salthouse, O., 93
Saltpeter, S., 141
Schneider, J. A., 4
Schoder, D., 107
semantic association tests, 112
semantic fluency, tests of, 65
semantic memory, 39
sensory impairment, as
    possible explanation for
    cognitive decline, 23
Sex Offenders Act (2003), 167
Sherman, E., 55
Sims, J. R., 144
simultanagnosia, 66
single-photon emission
    computed tomography
    (SPECT), 161–2
and distinguishing of
    Parkinsonian disorders
    from other disorders,
    98

Skoog, I., 149
sleep disorders, in DLB, 93
sleep disturbance
    reducing, 152
    relationship with dementia,
        8, 152
Slick, D., 55
small vessel disease (SVD), 75,
    76, 77, 78
Smith, J. S., 121
smoking, relationship with
    dementia, 150
Snowden, J. S., 111
social engagement, and
    reduction of dementia
    risk, 152
spatial processing, role of the
    dorsal stream, 38
Spector, A., 135
Spina, S., 61
Spinelli, E. G., 109
Steptoe, A., 9
story recall, 65
stroke, and incidence of
    VaD, 74
Stroop test, 66
structural imaging, CT and
    MRI, 159–60
Substance/Medication-
    Induced Major/Mild
    Neurocognitive
    Disorder, DSM-V
    diagnostic criteria, 125
Symptom Validity Tests, 54
synapse
    illustration of neuron and, 140
    meaning of, 34
synaptic pruning, 8

Takao, M., 92
TB v. KB and LH (Capacity to
    Conduct
    Proceedings), 171
temporal lobe, and processing
    of auditory
    information, 36
Test of Memory Malingering
    (TOMM), 54
Test of Premorbid Function
    (TOPF), 50, 53
testamentary capacity, 175
    Banks & Goodfellow, 175
    Clitheroe v. Bond, 175
    Kenward v. Adams, 175
The Awareness of Social
    Inference test
    (TASIT), 109

The End of Alzheimer's
    (Bredesen), 153
thiamine deficiency, see
    vitamin B1 (thiamine)
    deficiency.
tobacco use, relationship with
    dementia, 150
transient ischaemic attacks
    (TIAs), 76
transneuronal degeneration,
    meaning of, 34
traumatic brain injury, as risk
    factor for developing
    FTD, 106
Trembath, M. K., 7

Ulugut, H., 110

Van Damme, I., 124
vanishing cues, 132
vascular cognitive impairment/
    dementia (VCI/VaD)
    overview, 74
    case studies, 80–1
    cognitive profile, 77–8
    diagnostic criteria, 78–80
    genetics, 77
    imaging, role in diagnosis, 78
    life expectancy, 74
    neuropsychiatric signs, 78
    pathology, 75
    prevalence and incidence,
        74
    risk factors, 76–7
    VCI and Alzheimer's disease
        (mixed dementia), 75–6
    key points, 80
Velakoulis, D., 109
ventral stream, 38
    example of selective
        impairment to, 38
verbal fluency, tests of, 65
Villebrun, D., 121
vitamin B, 153
vitamin B1 (thiamine)
    deficiency
    and alcohol-related
        neurotoxicity, 123
    facilitating
        mechanisms, 123
    and Wernicke–Korsakoff's
        syndrome, 35, 122–3,
        125, 153
    links between Wernicke's
        encephalopathy,
        Korsakoff's syndrome
        and, 122

vitamin E, 153
Vogels, R. L., 23

Walterfang, M., 109
Warrington, E. K., 111
Wechsler Adult Intelligence
    Scale (WAIS), 48,
    49–50, 51–2, 53
Wechsler Memory Scale
    (WMS), 49, 51–2,
    53
Weigmann, C., 150
Wernicke, Carl, 122
Wernicke–Korsakoff's
    syndrome (WKS)
    case study, 127
    comparison with
        DAT, 126
    confabulation and, 124
    diagnostic criteria, alcohol-
        related and non-
        alcoholic variants, 125
    executive dysfunction
        and, 124
    neuroanatomy, 123–4
    neuropsychological
        assessment, 126
    prevalence, 121
    thiamine deficiency and, 35,
        122, 125, 153
    treatment, alcoholic vs
        non-alcoholic
        variants, 123
Wernicke's aphasia, 39
Wernicke's encephalopathy
    Korsakoff's syndrome
        and, 122
    thiamine and, 122, 123
Wijnia, J. W., 125–6
Williams-Gray, C. H.,
    88
Winter, L., 135
Wood, R., 171
Woods, B., 135
Woods, R. T., 135
Word Memory Test
    (WMT), 54
World Alzheimer Report
    2015, 1
Wu, M., 59

young-onset Alzheimer's
    disease (YOAD), 61

Zaccai, J., 90, 92
Zakzanis, K. K., 65
Zalesky, A., 34